Improvising Medicine

IMPROVISING
MEDICINE

An African
Oncology Ward in an
Emerging Cancer
Epidemic

JULIE LIVINGSTON

DUKE UNIVERSITY PRESS
Durham & London 2012

© 2012 Duke University Press
All rights reserved

Printed in the United States of America
on acid-free paper ∞
Designed by Jennifer Hill.
Typeset in Arno Pro by
Tseng Information Systems, Inc.

*Library of Congress
Cataloging-in-Publication Data appear on
the last printed page of this book.*

All photographs in this book by
the author, Julie Livingston.

In memory of Dikeledi Moloi

CONTENTS

In 2006 I returned to Botswana after an absence of some years, to begin research on a book about pain and laughter. On my first weekend back, a dear friend invited me for lunch at her home. She said she had been saving something for me, and she handed me a huge, flat, brown envelope. Inside were the CT scans and X-rays of her dead cousin, whom I had known long before as an energetic teenager. On the CT images, a massive tumor could be seen pushing through the colored slices of his head. She was unsure what to do with these pictures. It seemed wrong to throw them out, but they also were too upsetting to look at. Instead, she gave them to me, along with the story of his cancer. She told me she was sure I would find a way to put them to good use. In the coming days, other friends began to offer up cancer stories. Soon these stories led me to the pain and laughter I sought, but also to a great deal more.

This book is about a small cancer ward in Botswana. At this ward is a white, European doctor who tends to suffering, (mostly) black patients. The air is hot (in summer), and the sun bright. Some of the nurses are big, angelic mothers with wonderful rolling laughter. In the country next door, a murderous tyrant reigns. Uh oh. You might be worried already. She's written *that* book — the one Binyavanga Wainana warned us about in his deadly hilarious satire "How to Write about Africa." The book wherein some undifferentiated Africa lies marked by depravity, affliction, and beauty, awaiting the salvation of an equally unmarked "West."[1] But take heart, and please do not misread the chapters that lie before you. This is *not* a tale of white physicians come to save the poor Africans, if only they can overcome their ignorance and superstitions. We will not journey into "the diseased heart of Africa" to gaze at the spectacle while congratulating ourselves for caring.[2] There will be no hyenas or elephants, or even any big, red African sunsets. Africa will most certainly not be "pitied, worshipped, or dominated."[3]

Cancer, if you think about it, just doesn't lend itself to that kind of story. Cancer, like biomedicine itself, is neither an exclusively African problem, nor a particularly Western one. The problems of pain, death, illness, disfigurement, and care that lie at the heart of this book are basic human ones. But like all such experiences, they unfold on the ground in particular ways. Nor should cancer lend itself easily to the tales of redemption via biomedicine that make up the fantasies of global health. Thankfully, some cancers can be cured. Most, however, cannot. Oncology, like all domains of medicine, offers more than cure—it can help to extend the lives of patients, and it can palliate the afflicted, easing pain and discomfort. But these rewards are hard won if they come at all, gained through costly practices of poisoning, cutting, and burning. Any close look at oncology, as so many readers already know, necessarily means contemplating the deep ambiguities of biomedicine and our uncomfortable relationship with technological longing.

I myself cannot remember a time before cancer, before people I loved melted away and entered the agony of slow death, before surgical scars, and wigs, and bottles and bottles of pills. I also cannot remember a time before oncology. I was raised in the home of an oncologist who ran a cancer research lab. American, European, and Israeli cancer scientists and cancer doctors regularly visited our house, where oncology was a religion of sorts. Some of my dearest friends survived their cancers because of oncology, and for their continued presence I am immensely grateful. Yet, in the face of many deaths I have witnessed since childhood, I have also questioned oncology's rituals, its liturgy, and the excesses to which blind faith and desperation can lead. For many years, I noted its cultural, political, and economic power. I carried on in this manner until 1997, when, to my surprise, I found myself peeling apart cancer and oncology for the first time, so thoroughly interwoven had they been in my imagination.

In September of that year, for the first time in my life, I saw untreated, advanced cancer—that is, cancer without oncology. It was a horrible epiphany. I was in Botswana, visiting patients with a home-based care team, when I encountered a massive, florid growth that was killing a boy who slowly, silently writhed in agony. I stood stunned by the spectacle, unsure what I was seeing. My friend and co-worker, Dikeledi, whispered the word *cancer* in my ear, with a familiar gravity. I eventually saw many such scenes, and in the process came to understand that while cancer with oncology was awful, cancer without oncology could be obscene.

In the late 1990s in Botswana, these cancers seemed somehow ephemeral. Most people with an interest in healthcare in southern Africa were focused elsewhere—on HIV/AIDS. The politics of health were centered on gaining access to the new antiretroviral therapies (ARVs) that were suddenly extending the lives of people with HIV in the global north. Because such drugs were not available in Botswana, being far too expensive for the ministry of health to afford, many people wasted and died. What was to be done?

When I returned to Botswana for an extended stay in 2006, the situation had changed markedly. Antiretrovirals were now available, and the programs to distribute them were scaling up and continuing to enroll patients. But suffering, illness, and death had not disappeared, of course. Clearing away the cloud of AIDS revealed the landscape of cancers, which were attaching to a newly established oncology. But longing for oncology is not the same as longing for ARVs, as you will discover in this book.

The story before you necessitates the revelation of many personal matters and intimate details—a cancer ward is such a place where life is cut open, raw and exposed—but you won't find the X-rays my friend gave to me. They are simply too private. Similarly, you will not find photographs of cancer patients or their relatives. You will have to rely on my words and your imagination to grasp the humanity in the pages that follow.

ACKNOWLEDGMENTS

My greatest debt is to Dr. Alexander von Paleske, Matron Bertha Mapatsi, the entire nursing staff of Princess Marina Hospital's oncology department, and the many cancer patients and their relatives who opened their lives to me with unending patience during the most difficult of times. I also thank, in Botswana and Zimbabwe, Dr. Ahmed, Dr. Selthako, Dr. Ralefala, Dr. Zola, Dr. Chilume, Dr. Pietkar, Dr. Phutego, Dr. Kasese, Dr. Heunis, Dr. Gluckman, Dr. Hafkin, Dr. Ramagola-Masire, Dr. Hakuna, Dr. Vuli, and Dr. Gureja, who taught me a great deal about the practice of medicine. Patrick Monnaese, Dikeledi Moloi, and especially Bontsi Dikagamotse provided expert assistance during interviews. I am grateful to the Botswana ministry of health and Princess Marina Hospital for granting me permission to undertake this research.

Thatcher Ulrich accompanied me to Botswana, though it was profoundly disrupting to his own work and life. He gave me the time and space to write, and was a wonderful and generous sounding board. Hazel Livingston, too, was uprooted twice for the sake of this book; she has proven a terrific traveling companion. In Bulawayo, Mwaiti Sibanda and Alexander von Paleske took wonderful care of me, including organizing the loveliest Rosh Hashanah celebration for me that I can remember. In Gaborone, Kirsten Weeks opened her home and hosted me for over a month of deep conversation alternating with total hilarity. Also in Gaborone, Betsey Brada, in addition to being a terrific conversation partner and scrabble opponent, cared for me during a serious health crisis with the same sure hand she brings to all things. Michelle Schaan, Chris

Schaan, Isabella Schaan, and Patrick Monnaese made our stay on Kgwa-kgwe road much more fun.

This book is the product of a conversation sustained over the course of several years with my dear friend and intellectual comrade Steve Feierman. Many of the questions I ask here were initially his, and so, too, many of the answers. Steve has patiently read drafts and been my most consistent interlocutor since I began this research. I am immensely grateful to the Wissenschaftskolleg zu Berlin for giving us an entire year together in Berlin. In addition to Steve, the other members of the body-antibody group—Lynn Thomas, David Schoenbrun, and Nancy Hunt—have been extraordinarily generous and rigorous readers and listeners over the course of the research and writing, and I offer them my most heartfelt appreciation. There aren't words enough on this planet to thank Jennifer Morgan, brilliant scholar and beautiful, intuitive human being that she is, for all that she has contributed to this book, including but certainly not limited to the close reading she provided of the manuscript. João Biehl, Vinh-Kim Nguyen, Dietrick Niethammer, and Nancy Hunt read the entire manuscript and offered wonderful support and smart advice. Working with Ken Wissoker, of Duke University Press, has been a true joy, and I consider myself extremely fortunate to have him as my editor.

Robby Aronowitz read multiple chapters, and followed always with engaged conversations and fascinating questions. Keith Wailoo also read multiple chapters and provided expertise and encouragement. Work with Keith, Robby, and Steven Epstein on another book shaped my thinking here in important ways. Hansjörg Dilger offered me a place to first present what became the interlude here, "Amputation Day at PMH." The encouragement I received from him and from Kristine Krause, Nancy Hunt, Rijk van Dijk, and David Kyaddondo with regard to this material was invaluable. Sherine Hamdy asked tough questions with great warmth and kindness. Sharon Kaufman provided multiple comments on what is now chapter 6, "After ARVs, During Cancer, Before Death." Her clarity of mind and expertise were extremely helpful to me in sorting out my ideas, and I am grateful for her patience as I wrote and rewrote.

Rachel Prentice read several chapters and engaged me in long, fascinating conversations about phenomenology, ethics, and medicine that were true highlights of the writing process. Carolyn Rouse all at once grasped and clarified the underlying logic of the book for me, and suggested the title. Herman Bennett and Ann Fabian hatched this project in its embryonic form, sending me off to Botswana with crucial questions that sustained me through my research and writing. Seth Koven helped me conceptualize important stylistic and methodological questions. Randy Packard was generous, critical, and supportive as always. Paul Landau made sure I paid attention to laughter. From the beginning, Megan Vaughan, João Biehl, Stacey Langwick, and Mike McGovern asked all the right questions while offering the kind of continual faith and support in a humanist approach that I badly needed.

Rutgers, and especially the history department, continues to be a wonderful place to work and think, and I am thankful to have such great colleagues. During the writing of this book, I spent two wonderful years engaged in regular conversation with Indrani Chatterjee, Jan Kubik, and other members of the Vernacular Epistemologies Seminar at the Rutgers Center for Historical Analysis. I trust that Indrani and Jan both will recognize their significant influence on the finished product. Jasbir Puar, with whom I collaborated on a separate project, will also, I hope, recognize the many ways our regular conversations shaped my thinking here.

I am thankful to the many other people who read and commented on various drafts and exchanged ideas: Vincanne Adams, Kamran Asdar Ali, Joe Amon, Mia Bay, Alastair Bellany, Sara Berry, Betsey Brada, Allan Brandt, Tim Burke, Ed Cohen, Jennifer Cole, Barbara Cooper, Fred Cooper, Stefan Ecks, Harri Englund, Karen Feldman, Michael M. J. Fischer, Mary Fissell, Wenzel Geissler, Rene Gerrets, Clara Han, Gabrielle Hecht, Alison Isenberg, David Jones, Olivia Judson, Temma Kaplan, Fred Klaits, Seth Koven, David Kyaddondo, Pier Larson, Margaret Lock, Anne-Maria Makhulu, Harry Marks, Marissa Mika, Benson Mulemi, Herbert Muyinda, Iruka Okeke, Kris Peterson, Adriana Petryna, Mary Poss, Ruth Prince, Michael Ralph, Lesley Sharp, Bonnie Smith, Janelle Taylor, Susan Reynolds Whyte, Brad Weiss, Kay Warren, and Laurel Thatcher Ulrich.

Several chapters and the final revisions of this book were written in Berlin, at the Wissenschaftskolleg zu Berlin, amid an amazingly thoughtful group of people. In particular, Claire Messud, Hannah Ginsborg, Kamran Asdar Ali, Olivia Judson, Behrooz Ghamari-Tabrizi, Niklaus Largier, Albrecht Koschorke, Mike Boots, Iruka Okeke, Tanja Petrovic, and Elias Khoury showed me entirely new ways to think and write.

For true understanding and laughter in the bluest moments, which sometimes crept up on me while I was writing this book, I thank Annika Tamura, Megan Vaughan, David Schoenbrun, Lynn Thomas, Nicole Fleetwood, Herman Bennett, Olivia Judson, Jennifer Morgan, Claire Messud, Jasbir Puar, Stacey Langwick, Nancy Hunt, Steve Feierman, Betsey Brada, Alyssa Yee, Kate Gakenheimer, Jennifer Morgan, Robby Aronowitz, Karen Feldman, Vera Schulze-Seeger, and Paul Landau. I am especially grateful to Behrooz Ghamari-Tabrizi, brilliant mind, patient, generous soul, and avatar of care. He understood what I was doing and invariably knew how and why to make me laugh.

This book is dedicated to the memory of one very dear, departed friend, and to the too many loved ones lost over the years. It is also offered in deep celebration of those who are healed.

The Other
Cancer Ward

In the oncology ward of Princess Marina Hospital (PMH), Botswana's central referral hospital, a light breeze is blowing the curtains in the female side of the ward. It is that cool pause in the morning before the dry heat settles in for the day in Gaborone, Botswana's capital. Ellen is sitting up in her bed, dressed in her nylon, butterfly-print nightgown, retching into a vomitus—an enormous, lidded, stainless-steel basin. Piled on the stand next to her bed are cards, boxes of juice, bananas, and other gifts from relatives and friends. The two pairs of underpants and spare nightgown she laundered in the bathroom down the hall are draped across the headboard of her bed, drying. Next to her lies Lesego, age sixty, and a former teacher. With her enormous glasses perched on her nose, Lesego is silently reading her Bible. This is her fourth year as a cancer patient, and she is used to the rhythms of the ward. She knows that soon Tiny will come, rolling the metal breakfast cart through the aisle, pouring a tin or plastic mug of tea with milk and sugar for each patient, and dishing out plates of *motogo*, a sorghum porridge. It isn't a Tuesday or a Thursday, so there won't be a hard-boiled egg and tiny mound of salt.

Across the nursing desk in the men's side of the ward sits Roger, age twenty, whose left eye is swollen shut from a lymphoma. He is trying with little success to drink a small carton of strawberry-flavored Ensure (a nutritional supplement), as Mma T encourages him in that matter-of-fact, joking way that nurses so often use to cajole their patients. A few moments ago, he, too, was bent over his vomitus. Already he is melting away. Strangely enough, Roger's half-uncle, Mr. Mill, a white Motswana farmer with multiple myeloma, had vacated that same bed only the evening before Roger arrived. The ward is full right now, as usual, with twenty-one patients total—one extra bed has been crammed into the female side of the ward, the only ward in the hospital that refuses to house patients on the floor.

The cancer ward sits at the end of a corridor that is lined with long, narrow wooden benches. There patients and their relatives sit waiting to see the highly impassioned and, by all accounts, brilliant, if at times irascible, German oncologist, Dr. P. Some rose long before dawn for bus or ambulance rides from villages deep in the Kalahari Desert. Others arrive from nearby urban homes, or large towns in Botswana's southeast. Many will wait five or six hours or more for their turn in the clinic office with the hospital's lone oncologist, who not only attends to an average of twenty-five (but sometimes as many as forty) outpatient visits in the day, but also manages the ward, fills out paperwork (in triplicate with carbon sheets between the copies), administers chemotherapy, and performs his own cytology in the evenings. After he climbs onto a chair in a vain but unrelenting attempt to coax the highly improbable ward television set to life, he drives home, where he will finish the day's paperwork after eating dinner.

Formerly a lawyer in Frankfurt, and a disillusioned ex–Mugabe supporter, Dr. P was already in his mid-fifties when he came to Botswana from Zimbabwe, where he had practiced oncology at Mpilo Hospital in Bulawayo for fourteen years. Leaving wasn't easy. His wife, Mma S, remains in Zimbabwe, but visits Dr. P some weekends, during which she loads up her car with supplies no longer available back home. Mma S has been around the world and has lived abroad. She knows it is one thing to travel, another altogether to leave her country (and the private ultrasound practice she has built) and live as an African exile, a *lekwerekwere* (African immigrant or outsider). Come what may, Mma S has decided to stay in her home.

Dr. P also writes a column, strident in tone, for one of the Botswana newspapers, using the forum to lash out against white mercenaries, Rupert Murdoch, and corrupt African politicians. He is more than willing to stand up in the staff meeting and proclaim PMH a Potemkin village! But his respect for Botswana runs deep. His sometimes explosive temper and his bluntness—so out of place in Botswana—are by turns comedic, endearing, and infuriating to clinical staff, patients, and their accompanying relatives. Dr. P is chronically impatient and characteristically relentless in caring for his patients. Some days it seems the ward is running on the sheer force of his personality; occasionally it seems that it is running despite it. Each day he brings a crate of fruit to the clinic office, sharing bananas, grapes, peaches, plums, oranges, and apples, all in their season, with staff and visitors. He always wears a white coat in clinic. He enjoys nothing more than a joke made at his expense, except perhaps a political debate.

On one side of the corridor, opposite the clinic office, is the treatment room (also called the chemo room), with its sink and metal examination table. Various supplies, such as bags of IV saline and sterile dressing packs, are stored in this room, and occasionally the doctor uses this room to hold brief counseling sessions for the relatives of terminal patients, since end-stage prognoses are rarely discussed in front of the dying. Most important, chemotherapy is administered here, sometimes with three or four patients crammed in together on makeshift seating, their intravenous lines stretching like the legs of an octopus from a pole in the center of the tiny room. When one patient begins to vomit, the others often start heaving as well, and a nurse or the visiting ethnographer distributes pieces of paper towel and plastic bags. It is hot and stuffy in the treatment room, the air conditioner having broken long ago, but staff try to keep the doors shut, for the sake of the patients waiting on the benches. For some, even a peek into the treatment room or at the tubes of "the red devil" (doxorubicin, a chemotherapy drug) is enough of a mnemonic for the experience of chemo to bring on spontaneous waves of nausea and a panicky dread.

A decade ago the cancer ward was part of the Accident and Emergency Department of PMH. But the Botswana ministry of health predicted a rise in cancer and therefore refitted the observation wing of Accident and Emergency as the country's one and only cancer ward, bringing Dr. P on staff to oversee operations. Mma M, the ward matron, bore the loneliness of leaving her husband and children in order to study at an Australian university, becoming the first—and, until recently, the only—nurse in the national health system with specialized oncology training.

In addition, a small radiotherapy outpatient practice was developed across town, at the Gaborone Private Hospital (GPH). There, two radi-

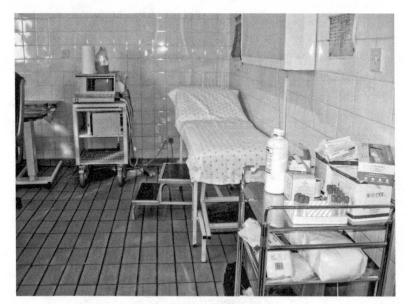

The clinic office and exam room.

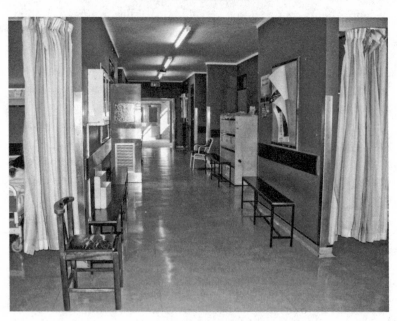

The hallway by the clinic.

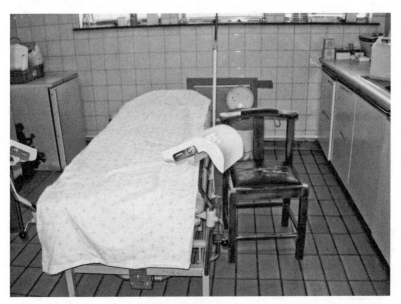

The chemotherapy and treatment room.

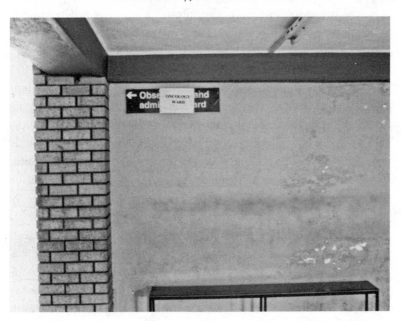

The entrance to the ward.

ation oncologists see public patients, whose treatments are paid for by the government and coordinated by PMH oncology. More recently, an oncologist was brought on placement through a partnership with the Chinese government to work in the medical wards of the only other tertiary hospital in the public health system: Nyangabwe, in Botswana's second city, Francistown.[1] Though some people do avail themselves of private doctors, particularly patients who receive medical insurance through their jobs, Botswana's system of universal care ensures that most people use the public system. As the hub of care and in coordination with these other sites, the PMH cancer ward remains the center of oncology in the country, and the only dedicated cancer ward.[2]

Improvising Medicine tells the story of this place—Botswana's oncology ward and its associated clinic—from its birth, in late 2001, to 2009. In the pages that follow we will observe patients, their relatives, and ward staff as a cancer epidemic rapidly emerges in Botswana, reflecting the surge in cancers across the global south. The stories of this ward dramatize the human stakes and the intellectual and institutional challenges of the cancer epidemic. They illustrate how care proceeds amid uncertainty in contexts of relative scarcity. They also offer fresh perspective on cancer medicine and illness experiences more broadly.

The argument I present is three-fold. First, improvisation is a defining feature of biomedicine in Africa. Biomedicine is a global system of knowledge and practice, but it is also a highly contextualized pursuit. Everywhere, doctors, patients, nurses, and relatives tailor biomedical knowledge and practices to suit their specific situations. In hospitals and clinics across Africa, clinical improvisation is accentuated.[3] Second, though cancer produces moments and states of profound loneliness for patients, serious illness, pain, disfigurement, and even death are deeply social experiences. Understanding cancer as something that happens *between* people is critical to grasping its gravity. In this respect, what I seek to make visible in PMH's oncology is not uniquely "African." Rather, it is an imperative that is often papered over or under threat in the techno-bureaucratic rituals of European or American wards, but which is nonetheless still there, beneath the surface: *care*.[4] I understand care within the context of debility and existential crisis as a form of critical "sociality based on incommensurate experience," to quote the anthropologist Angela Garcia.[5] By paying careful attention to care within the ward—

how it is imagined, enacted, and distributed, the moments in which it succeeds or fails — I present an anthropology of value that conjoins the biopolitical, the ethical, the social, and the human in medicine.[6]

Third, cancer in Africa is an epidemic that will profoundly shape the future of global health, raising fundamental policy, scientific, and care-giving challenges for Africans and the international community alike. Cancer is a critical face of African health *after* antiretrovirals (ARVs). As such, cancer experiences in the ward expose the unfortunate fact that biomedicine is an incomplete solution. It can simultaneously be redemptive and exacerbate existing health inequalities. In other words, there will be no quick techno-fix for African health. And yet biomedicine functions as a necessary, vital, palliative institution in a historically unjust world.[7]

The PMH oncology ward presents a compelling microcosm of twenty-first-century tertiary healthcare in southern Africa. The expertise that supports PMH oncology was assembled, in part, from African and European clinicians fleeing economic and political chaos elsewhere in Africa, Chinese and Cuban physicians brought in through bilateral development-assistance programs, and a group of Batswana nurses still reeling from the pressures of the AIDS epidemic. Its establishment was prompted by the fact that cancer was an anticipated byproduct of the first national public antiretroviral program in Africa, a program designed around a public-private partnership between the pharmaceutical industry, the Botswana government, and international philanthropy. Its promise is crafted out of the social, political, and demographic imperative to care for the sick that lies at the heart of Botswana's unusually robust social contract. Its form is marked by the contingencies, grittiness, and empirical challenges of providing high-tech medicine in a public hospital where vital machines are often broken, drugs go in and out of stock, and bed-space is always at a premium. Its patients are drawn from the full spectrum of Botswana's population, where "Bushmen" from the Kalahari lie in beds next to the siblings of cabinet ministers, and village grandmothers sit on chemo drips tethered to the same pole as those of young women studying at the university. And its cycles of promise and despair unite oncology's emphasis on hope with an African ethic of care that stresses continuous engagement, effort, and attempt.[8]

Taking a cue from Solzhenitsyn's remarkable novel *The Cancer Ward*, about a post-Stalinist ward in Tashkent, I present the ward as both a metaphor for and an instantiation of the constellation of bureaucracy, vulnerability, power, biomedical science, mortality, and hope that shape early-twenty-first-century experience in southern Africa. And as, quite simply, a cancer ward—a powerfully embodied social and existential space. In the process I will consider fundamental questions about the political and economic context of healthcare in Africa, the politics of palliation and disfigurement in the global south, the nature of decision making in clinical conditions of great uncertainty, and the social orchestration of hope and futility in an African hospital. I will contemplate the meanings, practices, and politics of care.

AN EMERGING EPIDEMIC

For all of its awfulness, cancer may sound like an esoteric distraction from more pressing concerns in African health. Yet epidemiologists have recently described cancer as a "common disease" in Africa.[9] This is part of a general trend in the so-called developing world, where more than half of all new cancer cases are already occurring, a situation made all the more acute given that developing countries deploy only a tiny fraction of the money spent on cancer globally.[10] And, as health experts have repeatedly stressed, the tide of cancer is rising steadily across Africa and the global south more broadly.[11] In Botswana's cancer ward this epidemiological shift is palpable. Dr. P wistfully remembers his first years in Botswana, when oncology beds lay empty and he cycled through other wards of the hospital actively searching for cancer patients to transfer to his ward. By 2006, when I first entered the ward, this scenario was difficult to imagine. Each year since the ward opened, patient queues have grown and pressure on bed-space has intensified. This trend persists despite programs developed to treat routine cases of the most common cancer, Kaposi's sarcoma (KS), at peripheral hospitals in the national network. But just how many cases of cancer are there, why are the numbers increasing, and what kinds of cancer are we talking about?

Cancer epidemiology is a complex business, given the expansive range of diseases under the cancer umbrella, as well as the need for laboratories with cytological and histopathological capacities to confirm diagnoses.[12] Africa has precious few cancer registries that feed into the International Agency for Research on Cancer (IARC) master registry of data collection. Basic medical certification is provided for only an estimated 13 percent of the deaths on the continent, and gathering accurate population figures is difficult in many sites. Botswana opened a cancer registry in 1999, but problems in staffing and coordination have greatly curtailed its ability, though these difficulties are now being sorted out.[13] Given the problems in collecting accurate data, most estimates of the burden of cancer in Africa are based on sentinel studies and on statistical models generated in a very few sites and then extrapolated to a broader population.[14] The figures I cite, taken from a two-part report by a team of leading cancer epidemiologists headed by D. Max Parkin, therefore are tentative ones. In addition, though this analysis is recent, it is based on data that are by now nearly a decade old, so these numbers almost certainly understate the current situation. They should be read with these caveats in mind.

In 2002, the year the PMH ward swung fully into action, there were an estimated 650,000 *new* cancer cases in Africa. Men and women, not surprisingly, suffered from slightly different cancers. For men, KS was the most common cancer, followed by cancer of the liver, prostate, bladder, lymphatic system (specifically non-Hodgkin's lymphoma), and esophagus. For women, cervical cancer took the lead, accounting for nearly a quarter of all female cancers, followed closely by breast cancer, which was responsible for nearly a fifth of all female cancers. After these came KS, liver cancer, non-Hodgkin's lymphoma, and ovarian cancer, in descending order. Significantly, epidemiologists also noted, "The importance of infectious disease in Africa . . . means that as many as 36% of cancers in Africa are infection-related, exactly double the world average."[15]

In the southern African region, where Botswana lies, the 2002 age-standardized incidence rates were the highest on the continent: 213.7 for males and 163.2 for females. These figures calculate the number of *new* cases per 100,000 persons in a year, based on a standardized age pyramid, which allows for comparison across populations with differing age distributions.[16] These rates were considerably lower than in North America, which had the highest incidence rates in the world: 398.4 for males and 305.1 for females. In North America, however, the comparatively high rates of cancer are partially accounted for by the proliferation of screening technologies that pick up early-stage asymptomatic disease. As Robert Aronowitz has argued, increasingly sensitive screening tests have resulted in what he calls "diagnosis creep" for some cancers, even as the rates for disease recurrence and fatality have remained stable.[17]

no asymptomatic cancer is reported

Southern Africa by and large lacks these screening programs, and as a result does not usually "count" cancers that have not progressed to the point where they produce symptoms.

Given this, perhaps equally telling is a comparison of the cancer mortality rates for these two regions: 158.5 (southern African males) versus 153.0 (North American males) and 106.3 (southern African females) versus 112.1 (North American females).[18] Mortality rates here represent the population's average risk of dying from cancer within the year. And so we can see that in 2002 while North Americans were much more likely to be diagnosed with cancer than southern Africans, they stood nearly equal chances of dying from the disease. For some population subgroups, the comparison is even starker. As Parkin and colleagues recently noted, "Even leaving aside the huge load of AIDS-related Kaposi's sarcoma [one of the most common cancers in these two sites], the probability of developing a cancer by the age of 65 years in a woman living in present day Uganda (Kampala) or Zimbabwe (Harare) is only about 30% lower than that of women in western Europe, and the probability of dying from a cancer by this age is almost twice as high."[19]

In Botswana partial epidemiological data, combined with anecdotal evidence and tallies from the ward and clinic, suggest that in PMH the most frequent cancers in men are KS, cancer of the esophagus, the prostate, head and neck, lung, and non-Hodgkin's lymphoma; in women cancer of the cervix, KS, breast cancer, non-Hodgkin's lymphoma, head and neck tumors, and cancer of the esophagus are most common. From this range of cancers, we can begin to discern two intersecting trends that combine to create a rising epidemic of cancer in the country.

Many of Botswana's cancer patients suffer from virus-associated cancers that are facilitated by HIV-related immunosuppression. These viral cancers include, but are not limited to KS (human herpes virus 8); genital cancers, of the cervix, vulva, anus, and penis (human papilloma virus); non-Hodgkin's lymphoma (Epstein-Barr virus, which is also associated with nasopharyngeal carcinoma and Hodgkin's disease); and head and neck tumors (often associated with human papilloma virus). A minority, but a significant number, of HIV patients will contract a virus-associated cancer either before being initiated on antiretroviral therapy or during the process of partial immune reconstitution. This should not be surprising. Experience in the United States has already shown that cancer and

HIV enjoy a troubling synergy, a dynamic underscored by the fact that three viral-associated cancers—KS, non-Hodgkin's lymphoma, and cervical cancer—serve as AIDS-indicator illnesses, which are complicated by the development of antiretroviral therapy. In 2003 program officials at the National Cancer Institute predicted the African cancer epidemic, and African oncologists and health planners, along with other members of the international oncology community, have been warning of rising incidence rates for some time.[20]

Before ARVs were available, many of Botswana's patients died *with* a cancer, but *from* other AIDS-related infections, while some died from rapidly growing cancers like high-grade non-Hodgkin's lymphoma. Since late 2001, when Botswana's ARV program began, however, many patients have survived HIV only to grapple with virus-associated cancers made all the more aggressive and difficult to treat by HIV co-infection. Botswana, where nearly a quarter of all adults have the HIV virus, is the site of the first public antiretroviral program in Africa, a model for programs now scaling up in neighboring countries. Yet, while ARVs are critically necessary and welcome in Botswana, they nonetheless expose the deadly relationship between cancer and HIV.

At the same time, the establishment of oncology services to assist patients with the new HIV-related cancers has helped to identify a significant population of patients with cancers not necessarily related to HIV—such as prostate, breast, esophageal, and lung cancer—who previously might have gone undiagnosed and untreated. The current cancer epidemic is deeply enmeshed with the HIV epidemic, but it is not only a subset of it. Breast cancers, for example, have long been present in the country but are now rising to a much greater level of recognition by both clinical staff and the general public. It is also quite likely that breast cancers are rising in overall incidence. Certainly, more and more women with breast cancer have been coming through the doors of PMH oncology. We cannot know the extent to which a long-standing burden of disease is now being unearthed through the expansion of services and public awareness, and the extent to which actual rates are rising. Most likely, it is a combination of the two. Over the past several decades Botswana has experienced rising rates of obesity, earlier onset of puberty for girls, lowered fertility rates, greater use of synthetic estrogens, and bottle feeding—all of which increase the risk of breast cancer. At the same time, new services mean that more women with breast lumps and wounds are being referred to PMH oncology for diagnosis.

BOTSWANA, CITIZENSHIP, AND UNIVERSAL CARE

Though historically overshadowed by tuberculosis, malnutrition, and, later, AIDS, cancer in Botswana predates the ward. Dr. Alfred Merriweather worked for over five decades in the country, becoming one of Botswana's most respected missionary doctors, as well as the first speaker of parliament in newly independent Botswana. Here, taken from his memoir published in 1999, is Merriweather's description of the female ward of the Scottish Livingstone Hospital in Molepolole, on his very first day in 1948, in what was then a twenty-four-bed mission hospital.

The elderly woman in the next bed was a pathetic case, one of very many I was to see in the years to come. She was in the late sixties very pale due to severe anemia, and she had experienced vaginal bleeding for over a year. She was asked how many children she had and replied, "I have had twelve but God has taken seven of them." We found the cervix of the uterus to be a friable mass of bleeding tissue eating its way into the vaginal wall and the bladder. She had advanced cancer of the cervix, the commonest cancer in Botswana, associated with early sexual activity and large families. . . . I always feel that this is one of the cruelest diseases a woman can have, for death is slow with many complications.

In the bed next to this cancer case was a young woman also with an inoperable cancer this time of the skin. She had a black swelling on the sole of her foot which had begun to ulcerate and in the groin a mass of enlarged glands. I had not seen such a tumor before and was told that it was a malignant melanoma, a very aggressive cancer. "I suggested we remove the ulcer on the skin as a palliative measure," said the doctor, "but like most of our patients she refused any surgery. She will only last a few weeks as the cancer is now widespread through her body."

Next to her was a woman, just skin and bone, probably in her mid forties. She had presented herself at the out-patient department with a history of having difficulty swallowing meat which started some months ago and gradually increased so that she could not swallow her staple diet of porridge. Latterly even to swallow water was a problem. She was starving to death. She had cancer of the gullet which, like cancer of the cervix I used to call a "cruel" disease. Such cases appear regularly in all our hospitals and the outlook is grim.[21]

Two decades after the scene that Dr. Merriweather recounts, in 1967, PMH opened to serve the new city of Gaborone and as the referral hospital for the estimated 630,000 citizens of a then newly independent Botswana. Over the next five years, 193 cancer patients received inpatient treatment in the wards, with cancer of the esophagus and the cervix still being among the most common forms of the disease. Dr. Johnson, the PMH surgeon at the time, felt certain that the cases he uncovered through a manual search of inpatient records represented an underreporting of the true extent of the disease.[22] Some patients refused admission and the recommended surgery, and many more, no doubt, never made their way to PMH in the first place. With most cancer patients who did come arriving with late-stage malignancies, many were denied admission because their disease was too advanced for treatment. At the time, PMH treated only a small fraction of the inpatient cancer cases in the country—nearly 1,500 between 1960 and 1972.[23] This would change in the years to come.

By the mid- to late 1990s, PMH was literally overflowing with patients. But the cancer ward was yet to open, and neither the English term *cancer* nor the Setswana term *kankere* were in common use. In those years I often saw cancer patients in the context of my research or during my leisure time, both of which took me into private homes. I sat with one friend while she sobbed for hours about the impending death of her only son, age five, from leukemia. He had recently returned from South Africa, swollen and bruised from several months' treatment at Chris Hani Baragwanath Hospital. Located in Soweto, it was the largest hospital in the world and had served Africans under apartheid. His grandmother had gone with him, sleeping each night on the floor next to his bed, while his mother remained in Botswana to work. Another friend's mother lay slowly dying of ovarian cancer on a mattress on the floor of her crowded two-room house. One time I accompanied staff from the clinic in the village where I lived to bring a packet of ibuprofen to a teenage boy lying on a mattress on the veranda of his home; his knee was swollen to impossible proportions from a bone cancer, a stunning spectacle that underscored the impotence of our small plastic bag of pills. His mother and aunt appeared to watch his every breath, as his agony suspended time.

In the 1980s and 1990s, before the ward was built, some cancer patients were sent to Zimbabwe or South Africa, where the Botswana government paid for them to receive oncology treatment in public hospitals. Many were not diagnosed until their disease was so advanced that they did not qualify for treatment referral. In other cases patients or their relatives decided not to pursue the prospect of referral abroad. In the 1990s, because of HIV, many Batswana were dying horrible deaths despite hospital care, and confidence in the biomedical system was flagging.[24] No doubt many of the relatives of these cancer patients suspected, quite often correctly, that even if their patients made the arduous journey to a foreign hospital, they might die anyway, but would also suffer as a result of being far from the comforts of home and family.

Even now, the government continues to send Batswana cancer patients to South Africa for specialized care unavailable in Botswana. Each week a government van brings women with cervical cancer for brachytherapy (internal radiation) and young patients with leukemia for induction or consolidation chemotherapy, which requires isolation conditions that are impossible to obtain at PMH. And many Batswana continue to look to South Africa as a place with more sophisticated and powerful medicine than is available in their own country. The ministry of health, will not, however, pay for other, more expensive treatments with lower likelihood of success, like bone marrow or organ transplantation, despite their availability in South Africa. For the state, achieving the greatest good for the greatest number sometimes means pushing back against the imperative of what the medical sociologist Mary-Jo DelVecchio Good has called the "biotechnical embrace."[25]

While Batswana still travel for care in South Africa, and indeed many patients look longingly across the southern border, Zimbabwe, to the northeast, presents a different story, one that throws Botswana, its history, and PMH oncology into relief. In December 2006, when Beauty's voice became hoarse and her throat painful and swollen, she and her husband feared the worst. Her laryngeal cancer had been in remission since 2000, when she was treated at Mpilo Hospital in Bulawayo. This time when she fell ill, her local primary hospital referred her south, to PMH. Though it was their first time in the ward, when they arrived Beauty and her husband found familiar faces. Dr. P discovered his own handwriting on her Mpilo discharge cards and called Dr. K., who had handled her initial radiation treatments, for a lunch-hour consult. Even though Beauty

Government interference [handwritten margin note]

and her husband had traveled south to Gaborone and PMH, rather than northeast to Bulawayo and Mpilo Hospital, she experienced a surprising continuity of care when the recurrence was unfortunately confirmed and treatment began.

A few years after Dr. P decided to leave Mpilo Hospital and head to PMH, he was joined in Gaborone by a Zimbabwean radiation oncologist, Dr. K, who had trained in Cuba and then worked with Dr. P at Mpilo for many years. By late 2003, the political and economic situation had become highly unstable in Zimbabwe, so Dr. K reluctantly crossed the border to join Dr. H, a white South African radiation oncologist, in running the new radiotherapy practice at the Gaborone Private Hospital. This was the first and at present is still the only site for external radiation in the country; public patients were sent there on the government's dime. Unlike the public hospital, the private hospital was lucrative, with radiation treatments costing the government up to thousands of dollars per patient.

Dr. K and Dr. H both drove BMWs and wore much nicer shoes than did Dr. P, who was known to use a stapler to repair his sandals. This gave Dr. P, who came of age as a left-wing protester in 1968 in Germany, some deep ideological satisfaction. Before lunch most days, Dr. K or Dr. H came to PMH for a quick consult to coordinate care for the government radiotherapy patients. Eventually Dr. Z, a Congolese pathologist, and Dr. G, a Liberian surgeon at Mpilo, would also make their way from Bulawayo across to PMH. And so Dr. P, the lone hematologist and oncologist at the hospital, found himself consulting with a cluster of colleagues with whom he had worked in the heyday of social medicine in Zimbabwe. Unfortunately, Botswana's gain was Zimbabwe's loss—something both Dr. P and Dr. K felt acutely. No lunchtime consult was complete without a brief exchange of news about Zimbabwe.

Botswana is unique in the southern African region (indeed, the continent) for its steady development trajectory, stable democracy, and system of functioning social-welfare programs, including its national healthcare program. At independence from British colonial rule, in 1966, Botswana was a deeply impoverished labor reserve serving South African industry, surrounded on all sides (but for the tiny Zambezi River crossing into Zambia) by institutionally racist colonial states. Since then, the discovery of vast diamond wealth and prudent investment by a stable, democratically elected government have meant rising standards of living,

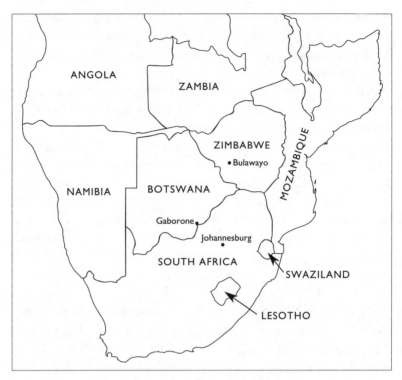

Map of Botswana in the region.

as well as significant investment in primary healthcare, clean water, nutrition, and infrastructure. Botswana's path to middle-income status was not some accident of history. For over four decades, Botswana's political leadership has proven remarkably adept, patient, and forward thinking in charting the course of development, stability, and peace under challenging circumstances.

Perhaps the most challenging circumstance has been the HIV epidemic, which wounded Botswana to its core. For about a decade, beginning in the mid-1990s, Botswana had the highest rate of HIV infection in the world. Human resources were devastated as the young sickened and died, and vast resources had to be redirected into healthcare at the household as well as the government levels. The AIDS epidemic and its attendant illnesses and deaths posed moral crises for Batswana, and a tremendous amount of soul-searching took place.[26] Now, with nearly a quarter of the adult population infected, HIV continues to pose significant challenges, but much has been learned, even if many dear friends have been lost.[27]

Healthcare (including oncology) is provided as a public good for citizens under a program of universal care. Most notably, Botswana has not accrued foreign debt, and so has been spared the predations of structural adjustment. Botswana accepts advice and assistance from others, but it is also a nation that makes its own decisions and speaks its own mind when it feels it appropriate. The pioneering ARV program was established through a partnership with the Gates Foundation and Merck pharmaceuticals, eventually expanding to include the contributions of Bristol-Myers Squibb, Harvard University, the President's Emergency Plan for AIDS Relief (PEPFAR), and the Global Fund. But the ministry of health has played the central role in dictating the terms of this arrangement, running the program within (as opposed to alongside) the national health system.[28]

As a result, Batswana do not have to grapple with the heart-wrenching dilemmas or intense economic pressures of unequal access to life-saving therapies like ARVs or oncology that abound elsewhere on the continent.[29] The privatization of public health across Africa has had a devastating effect on healthcare, a fact that erupts in the ward each time a noncitizen arrives for treatment and must bring cash to cover the costs of care.[30] Often these patients come because care is unavailable at home, as in 2008, when Zimbabwean patients arrived at PMH reporting that there was *nothing* in the hospitals in Bulawayo—*not even a panado* (paracetamol or acetaminophen).

None of this is to suggest that Botswana is without economic or political inequalities or tensions, which often map onto minority ethnic status, gender inequalities, class politics, or regional economic differences within the country.[31] These are significant problems, though they remain somewhat outside the scope of this book. Nor does it mean that all Batswana are wealthy. They are not. While the state has invested in public infrastructure and safety nets, the gap between rich and poor has also grown steadily since independence, and just under a third of the population lives below the poverty line.[32] Many who appear to be gainfully employed are deeply in debt to Botswana's thriving credit economy.[33] There may be Mercedes-Benzes parked in the lot at PMH during visiting hours, but there are also many patients who have real trouble borrowing the funds necessary for bus fare to their clinic appointments.

Nor can one be certain about the future availability of healthcare. Because of the global economic crisis, the Botswana government warned, in 2009, that it might be unable to enroll new patients on ARVs after 2016.[34] In 2011 the country was rocked by a massive public-sector strike, in which many health workers walked off the job to protest their conditions of employment. Nonetheless, having built an extensive primary-care system essentially from scratch throughout the 1970s, 1980s, and 1990s, the Botswana government has prioritized the expansion and improvement of access to tertiary care in recent years. Thus, new services like oncology have been developed within PMH, one of only two tertiary-care centers in the public healthcare system, as stop-gap measures while new broader institutional capacities are being developed.

Plans for construction of a more up-to-date and capacious national referral hospital are now under way, as part of the establishment of the country's first medical school. This medical school will enroll citizens of Botswana, thus developing a cadre of local medical and research expertise. Because of long-standing national policy, nearly all the nurses in the national health system are Batswana. But at the time of this writing, the vast majority of doctors, particularly specialists, are not. There are some notable exceptions, of course, like Dr. O, an extremely skilled Motswana maxillofacial surgeon, who also ran the dental clinic, or Dr. R, who is pioneering a women's health center through a partnership between PMH and the University of Pennsylvania. Other younger Batswana medical officers—like Dr. C and Dr. S, both of whom worked many months in oncology during their rotations through the various wards of PMH— have gone abroad for specialty training with plans to return. But for now, most specialists and many medical officers ("residents" in American terminology) tend to come from other parts of Africa and from Europe, Asia, and North America.[35] And for the foreseeable future, PMH remains Botswana's hospital of resort.

CANCER

Perhaps no disease is so iconic for and familiar to American and European readers as cancer. This unfortunate fact provides the opportunity for readers from these places to know Botswana and its patients as part of a broader community of biomedical practice and bodily experience. In one sense *Improvising Medicine* traces a remarkably familiar tale of cancer as experienced outside the elite oncology centers like Dana Far-ber or Sloan Kettering. The PMH ward will be instantly recognizable to anyone who has spent time with cancer. Just as in American or European hospitals, the therapies are intensive and aversive, and the cure often elu-sive, but hope animates the daily dynamics. Patients often feel alienated and intimidated by hospital bureaucracy. But individual clinicians, fellow patients, and especially nurses have the power to humanize the illness experience. Errors in this hospital are common, just as they are in bio-medical institutions throughout the world.[36] Cancer patients and their caregivers in Botswana face the same existential, temporal, and moral questions that trouble cancer patients everywhere: the temporal urgency of oncology; the deeply aversive yet potent nature of therapeutic inter-ventions: chemotherapy, surgery, and radiation; the uncertainty of the future; the threat of nihilism.

Yet amid all this familiarity, this sameness, lie critical questions of re-sources that are more easily revealed in a public hospital in a middle-income country, where triage is not left to market forces (masked through the oracular bureaucracy of health insurance), but rather must occur within an explicit pragmatics of universal access. Even within the ethos of collective compassion evidenced in robust medical citizenship, cure, despite its elusiveness, is often given precedence over a more ex-pansive form of care. The PMH ward lacks the amenities—the power-ful anti-emetics, the morphine pumps and fentanyl patches, the breast reconstructions, the professional counseling and informational litera-ture—meant to smooth the rough edges of oncology, one of biomedi-cine's most brutal, if hopeful domains of practice.

Oncology is predicated on a temporal urgency. As any patient (not only in Botswana) will tell you, a cancer diagnosis hurls one into a thera-peutic pipeline at great speed. Dr. P recognizes that cancer patients can-not wait to be seen, without serious consequences. At PMH he is com-mitted to seeing all the cancer patients who require attention on the day they arrive, rather than booking appointments with waiting times of weeks or even months for the newly diagnosed. He could send the patients away and ration his time so that his workload would be reason-able, perhaps fifteen patients a day. But then those patients who would be waiting to see him would only be getting sicker, their prognosis more tenuous, their pain more profound, and success even more elusive. "I won't save myself any work in this way unless the patient dies in the meantime while waiting for their appointment, and this is utterly unacceptable," he told me. Yet, since there is only one oncologist, the temporal urgency means that each patient gets little time to discuss their problems with the doctor, and so the humanistic side of oncology is, unfortunately, greatly curtailed.

Questions of therapeutic intervention and futility also take on a different tone here. The desire to intervene in cancers, to extend life, to palliate through surgery, radiation, or chemotherapy is fueled by a daily look at the natural course of disease progress. A context, as in the United States, wherein many cancers are treated aggressively when they are still microscopic or asymptomatic engenders a public conversation about iatrogenic effects of aggressive therapies and their value. In Botswana, where florid, disfiguring growths and horrible pain drive patients with late-stage cancers into the clinic for diagnosis each day, the palliative nature of oncology for the terminally ill is more clearly recognized as a public good, and stage 0 cancers or precancerous growths are not part of the popular experience of the disease.

The clinical science that drives therapy is also familiar, if radically pared down. In Botswana, perched on the periphery of the metropolitan oncological imagination, we see cancer diagnosis performed in an institution where histology is uncertain, where crucial technologies often break and cannot be repaired for weeks or months on end. This is a hospital that lacks a magnetic resonance imaging (MRI) machine, mammography, and endoscopy, where the lone oncologist performs his own cytology on a donated microscope after clinic hours, and where genetic screening and nuclear medicine are impossible. Cancer medicine lies at the cutting edge of the biomedical enterprise. Yet cancer medicine as it is practiced in Botswana, in many ways a best-case scenario for African public health and clinical medicine, bears a strange relationship to the research agendas of academic medicine and the private pharmaceutical industry. Oncology here does not match "evidence-based medicine" or "best practices" as developed in the West. The technical, biological, and social conditions of medical care in Botswana differ greatly from those from which knowledge and standards of care are derived. Dr. P must continually improvise and work empirically as he treats patients with tuberculosis *and* cancer, late-stage presentations, and HIV co-infections in a context that lacks some of the drugs, equipment, expertise, and diagnostic technologies that are standard in Western hospitals.

The existential angst and reflection among patients and their loved ones trace common threads. Yet the content of patient expectations, the forms of prognostication, and the ethics of clinical decision making follow slightly different logics than the American model, which privileges patient autonomy, presumes a baseline familiarity with cancer and its trajectories, and ponders the ambiguities of technologies like feeding tubes and respirators. The HIV/AIDS epidemic in Africa has already generated tremendous debate over biomedical ethics. The cancer epidemic raises a new set of questions—about rationing, prognostication, and futility. For example, here is a typical scenario: five patients each need between four and six units of platelets. Yet the hospital blood bank only has five units total to dispense. How is Dr. P to decide how to distribute the platelets? Should each patient receive at least one unit? Or should all units go to the neediest case? The one with the best prognosis? Should the Mma Kgabo, who has failed to show up for two scheduled rounds of chemotherapy, be denied a share of the precious platelets as punishment for her "noncompliance"? Should Mr. Mill, whose prognosis is bleak, be denied platelets, even though he is the only patient actively bleeding? I will grapple with a range of such questions and also describe how relatives and clinical staff negotiate with one another to locate therapeutic futility for the dying in a setting that lacks bed-space, hospice care, and adequate counseling resources.

The PMH oncology ward is an improvised setting. It leaves much to be desired, as its staff readily acknowledge. Examining processes of making do, tinkering, and ad-libbing help us to better understand the nature of biomedicine in Africa and the work of African healthcare workers, for whom improvisation is inevitably the modus operandi. Yet the story of this ward is not only one of cultural difference or of poverty, but also of innovation and care, and of therapeutic futility. Batswana cancer patients and oncology staff are part of a global therapeutic community—as they improvise, they also dislodge some of the master narratives of cancer in the global north. This book calls into question some of the prescriptive, heroic narratives and basic assumptions about illness, death, hope, and medicine that many American patients, their clinicians, and family members often take for granted. Like David Rieff's recent memoir about Susan Sontag's final year of cancer, or Lucy Grealy's *Autobiography of a Face*, this book doesn't offer easy answers as to how families, patients, or practitioners should respond to grave illness. Nor does it shy away from the microprocesses of biomedical care—the nasogastric tubes, bone-marrow aspirates, wound care, and the suctioning of tracheostomies. Rather than portraying these routinized procedures as minor details, subordinated to the main events of diagnosis and cure, this book shows how cancer experience, hope, and futility are built up through such uncomfortable practices. By stepping outside of the familiar contexts in which heroic narratives, prostheses, pink ribbons, and invocations of cutting-edge research sanitize cancer experiences in the popular imagination, readers will find new ways to contemplate what it is to be seriously ill, extremely uncertain, and seeking relief.

A reminder. The cancer ward is a dramatic place animated by pressing existential concerns and aversive bodily experiences. But among the dramatic deaths, the arguments, the sudden crises, the curious events, and the quiet tears, it is also a tedious and boring place. In the clinic Dr. P sees patient after patient after patient. He performs fine-needle aspiration after fine-needle aspiration, breast palpation after breast palpation. The same blood work and then chemo regimen are ordered over and over again for the KS patients. Nurses and nursing assistants must fill out endless paperwork and computer forms and must routinely translate the same basic explanations and instructions. They must suction tracheostomy after tracheostomy, change diaper after diaper, and make and remake beds. Patients and relatives must spend the better part of a day sitting on the benches, clutching small pieces of cardboard with numbers written in magic marker to establish their places in the queue. To make matters worse, many patients cannot eat before their appointments, because they either lack the money to purchase a meal, or fear the nausea that will follow their treatments. Some cannot afford to waste money on a meal they are certain to vomit up. And so they spend these waiting hours simultaneously bored, anxious, and hungry. In the chemo room, syringes are lined up, drugs pushed, and the patient queue moved through as names are called.

For patients who are staying in the ward for days or weeks at a time, there is no working television, nor are there magazines or books to break up the long days. Patients who are ambulatory might walk outside and sit in the shade, or go to purchase juice or snacks or cell phone airtime from the small, corrugated-iron tuck shops that line the hospital parking lot. But aside from these limited diversions, there is not much to occupy patients or to link them to the outside world except for visiting hours:

Mindset effects

7–7:30 AM, 1–2 PM, 4–5:30 PM, and 7–7:30 PM. Many patients have relatives and friends who go to great lengths to be at their bedsides during these brief opportunities to visit. But many others have come to the ward from villages and towns many kilometers away, and their relatives may lack the time or money to visit often (or at all). Many patients are simply too sick to be bored, but they still might be homesick. Chatting with the nurses or the relatives visiting a patient in a neighboring bed or receiving a brief call or text on their cell phone may be their only links to the lives from which they have come. It is very difficult to appropriately convey this tedium in writing. In the pages that follow, I spend more time describing moments of crisis and action, than those of tedium and loneliness. But as you read I ask you to remember the many hours you yourself have no doubt spent waiting, sometimes for unpleasant or worrisome experiences, in highly bureaucratic and uncomfortable government institutions. Recall your own boredom in repeatedly performing the same monotonous tasks. Or think about the nights you have spent away from home knowing that life there was going on without you. And know that these kinds of experiences, too, are fundamental to cancer everywhere in the world.

THE METHOD, THE WRITING

The chapters that follow are based on intensive ethnographic research and are built on my long-standing knowledge of and engagement with healthcare and bodily vulnerability in Botswana.[37] During my work in Botswana—from November 2006 through May 2007, from June to July 2008, and in May 2009—I was granted privileged access to Botswana's oncology ward and clinic.[38] There I met patients, their relatives, and clinical staff as an American researcher and professor studying the nature of cancer medicine and care in the country, and as someone with a particular interest in questions of pain and palliation.

My methods were ethnographic, which means I spent many hundreds, if not thousands of hours observing and taking careful notes, and also participating in the daily activity of the ward. Thankfully, I was never a cancer patient at PMH, so my participation was inherently partial. I cannot fully understand the ward from the position of someone lying in one of the beds. Nor was I a doctor or nurse charged with performing the skilled and difficult work of oncology. But this does not mean that I did

recognizes her situation is not the same

not participate—only that my participation was shaped by my abilities and limitations. I shadowed the hospital's doctors, the nurses, and nursing assistants as they performed their daily tasks.

While staff in PMH oncology worked hard, the volume of patients created significant labor pressures, and it quickly became impossible to merely sit by and observe. I often accompanied patients to radiology or to consultations with specialists in other parts of the hospital, acting as a combined porter and liaison—helping to clarify why Dr. P was sending them for consult. I drove patients across town (often in Dr. P's car) to consultations at GPH, in order to save them the trouble, discomfort, and expense of a taxi or bus. I ran errands, often carrying drug orders to the pharmacy and syringes of cytotoxics back to the treatment room. I stood by during procedures as an extra pair of hands. For example, as patients underwent invasive diagnostic procedures (lumbar punctures, bone-marrow aspirates, etc.), I would sometimes help to hold them steady. Or I would assist a nurse cleaning a wound by helping to hold instruments or supplies that she could not touch while maintaining her sterile field. One patient who came regularly for transfusions would request that I come to hold her hand while the needles were inserted painfully into inguinal veins. Others wanted me to sit with them, maintaining eye contact, while they suffered the panic of respiratory distress beneath their plastic oxygen masks. While I sat in the clinic taking notes, patients, relatives, and staff often drew me into their diagnostic and prognostic conversations as a linguistic and cultural translator, given my knowledge of Setswana language, Tswana medicine, and biomedicine. Other times patients or relatives would use me as a sounding board. They recognized that I, unlike the busy staff, was someone who had more time to answer questions about the purpose of various technologies or about the nature of cancer, to listen to their existential angst, and to provide encouragement or at least recognition of the challenges of their predicament.

In addition to research in the ward, I worked in other domains of PMH in order to better situate cancer care, and questions of pain and palliation, within the larger institution. On occasion, I was present during the night or weekend shift in obstetrics and gynecology, or on the medical wards. There I had a small taste of the alternating exhaustion and adrenaline-fueled emergency response that the medical officers and nurses face as they regularly rotate through night duty. I attended rounds and staff meetings in the medical wards and in obstetrics and gynecology, and sat with two of the hospital radiologists who patiently showed me how to identify metastases on X-rays. In the evenings I viewed slides with Dr. P, who doubled as the hospital cytologist, learning the rudiments of this diagnostic vision. I observed the colposcopy clinic with Dr. T, at that time the head of gynecology, where suspected cervical cancers were diagnosed. I visited some patients in their village homes or in the interim home, a twenty-bed dormitory where ambulatory patients resided while undergoing their several-week-long radiotherapy treatments. There I conducted thirty-five interviews, in Setswana and English, with patients about their cancer experiences. I also deepened my extant knowledge of Tswana medicine through interviews with local healers, some of whom I had worked with during previous research on the history of debility and care.

In addition, I sat briefly on a palliative-care task force organized by the ministry of health. I accompanied Dr. P on a small plane to a peripheral hospital in the southwestern corner of the Kalahari to do oncological outreach. I attended rounds and clinic in a provincial hospital on several occasions and sat in the HIV clinics in various sites observing cancer referrals in creation. This ethnographic and interview work is enriched by historical research that locates African oncology and transnational oncology in a longer time frame, as part of the necessary background story of the ward.

In moving from the private homes and public spaces of village and town life, which comprised my previous research, and entering the cancer ward, I was practicing a form of "hospital-based ethnography." In order to understand how biomedicine is contextualized, it helps to spend time in its core institutions, hospitals.[39] Ethnographers recognize that the hospital is an intensive space where critical moral, political, and social questions arise regularly and with great urgency, and where broader political, social, and moral forces in society can be witnessed in a condensed fashion.[40] In other words, this ethnography describes oncology as a set of grounded practices occurring within a particular infrastructural, social, and epidemiological setting, rather than as a therapeutic ideal or model emerging out of cutting-edge research. I do not question evidence-based medicine or standards of care that emerge from careful metropolitan research; instead I witness how staff at PMH need to adapt this knowledge to their institutional setting like a round peg to a square hole. At the same time, this ethnography uses the limited stage of the ward as a venue to contemplate the broader meanings of care in twenty-first-century southern Africa. In order to protect the privacy of the patients whose stories are told here, I have changed their names and at times altered certain distinguishing details about them, while retaining the inherent logic of their medical and social specificities.

This book is written in the first person, but this is not a journey of self-discovery. Instead I keep myself in the scene because my presence in the situations described undoubtedly shaped what happened, and to write myself out of the text in the language of dispassionate science or journalistic voyeurism would be misleading. I wrote in the first person to be a bridge between different kinds of readers as well.[41] When I did ethnographic research in private homes, amid Tswana healers, and in village clinics in Botswana in the 1990s, I frequently recognized that everyone in the room except me understood what was happening. Life was brimming over with puzzles, and I was confused. Over many months, I groped my way toward enough social and cultural understanding to at least begin to grasp the depths of experience flowing around me. My research on cancer was quite different.

As I sat in the oncology clinic and ward with my black notebook and pen, I did not have this sense of puzzlement. Instead, I often felt like I was the only person in the room who really understood what was going on: the only one who knew enough about oncology or biomedical technologies (though far, far less, of course, than did Dr. P), enough about the hospital (though far, far less, of course, than Mma M or the other nurses), enough about Tswana medicine and forms of embodiment (though far less, of course, than many Batswana), enough about the intense challenges of care-giving in patient homes (though far less, of course, than most accompanying relatives), enough about the frustrations, pains, and fears of chronic illness and disfigurement (though far less than many PMH cancer patients) to perceive the miscommunications, the layers, the complexities of the daily dramas that unfolded in this clinical space. I felt like I had a holistic perception (albeit a somewhat superficial one) that transcended the intense, yet partial knowledge of everyone else. Of course, this hubris was often proven wrong: sometimes my assumptions were totally incorrect, and social or biological or institutional processes unfolded in ways that underscored my ignorance. Nonetheless, writing in the first person lets me convey some of this plurality of perspectives—to help you see this ward as a social space, a place where different kinds of knowledge, concerns, people, and entities combine to shape the experiences of very sick people and their caregivers.[42]

Lastly, this book is written in the first person because I hope to be a tool, a conduit through which you, the reader, can glean some dimension of the ward in a phenomenological sense. In other words, this book is concerned with forms of consciousness or knowledge that exceed the cognitive—forms that are sensory, bodily, affective. As my friend Ed likes to say, "You know more than you think," and this is a good way to understand phenomenology.[43] Experiences in this cancer ward underscore the extent to which phenomenology can be rendered social. For example, it is one thing to say that Botswana is a very small place and that at times staff in the ward will find themselves unexpectedly treating friends, relatives, or acquaintances who are cancer patients. It is another to experience, as I did on a few occasions, the sinking *feeling* one has on looking up from one's task to see a friend unexpectedly walk into the clinic as a newly diagnosed cancer patient, even while one tries to ensure that feeling is not conveyed on one's face. It is one thing to read that cancer wounds can be necrotic, and quite another to make sure to chat with a patient while holding the plastic bag into which his or her dead tissue is being deposited. My own experiences were greatly diluted from those of the nurses, doctors, relatives, and, most important, the patients. But throughout I include excerpts from my field notes to convey some of this quality. I wrote my field notes continuously throughout my time in the ward each day, whenever a free moment arose. In the evenings I reviewed them, adding details I remembered but couldn't elaborate on given the time pressures on the ward. Later I typed the notes into my computer, cleaning them up grammatically and occasionally making parenthetical connections that became clear to me as I reread them. I have placed quotations around all speech. Where I am certain I have someone's words verbatim, I have offered an asterisk to indicate as much. Where I am less certain that I have the exact phrasing, I do not. These field notes, therefore, give greater proximity to the ethnographic moment, but they are a mediated, not a raw product.

Some of the writing in this book is quite graphic, but that is necessary. Disturbing bodily experiences are foundational to patient experiences and biomedical practices of cancer. It may be unpleasant or even frightening to read about rotting flesh or about the process of shoving a flexible tube up a patient's nose, forcing him to swallow it so that he may be

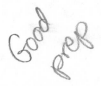
Good prep

fed. But cancer consists of such experiences. Their details are not gratu-
itous for the reader any more than they are for the patient. One strength
of ethnography as a mode of writing lies in its ability to communicate
these details as they are emplotted in experiences of illness and care.
These details help to establish the stakes of illness and medical care, the
disorienting immediacy of bodily experiences, and the forms of bodily
consciousness that are produced through profound illness and practices
of care. Nonetheless these are very intimate matters, and therefore I have
taken great pains to include only those graphic accounts I think are absolutely essential to your understanding of the experiences at hand.

TWO

Neoplastic Africa

Mapping Circuits of
Toxicity and Knowledge

On 20 May 2009, months after the Zimbabwean government had appealed for international assistance in responding to an outbreak of cholera, twenty-eight new cases and one cholera death were reported. By then, as the epidemic was beginning to wane, nearly 100,000 people had fallen sick and over 4,000 had died, according to official reports.[1] The vast majority of the country had been affected, and the disease had crossed borders, with cases reported in Botswana, Mozambique, Zambia, and South Africa.

The cholera epidemic in Zimbabwe was horrifying in human terms and dangerous in its rapid, far-reaching spread, and it offered stark political testimony of just how far the Mugabe regime had allowed sanitation, water, and healthcare infrastructure—in fact, all vestiges of the social contract—to erode. The nineteenth-century narrative of cholera was yet again revived, through the twenty-first-century misery of Zimbabwe's now great unwashed and the rapaciousness of the Zimbabwean political elite. For all that it was unimaginable, the epidemic was all too familiar, and a predictable global-health apparatus of water-purification tablets, medicines, doctors, epidemiologists, and supply trucks sputtered into action.

But on that same day—20 May 2009—there was another Zimbabwean death, this one across the border in Gaborone, Botswana. It wasn't cholera that killed Lovemore Makoni. The disease that killed him, though equally appalling, was much more common. Yet, ironically, that disease was largely absent from Western images of African health and illness. Lovemore lay in the medical ward of PMH, short of breath, wracked with pain and panic. Mr. Makoni, a barman at a local club, had cancer (KS) in his lungs. He urgently needed chemotherapy, which fortunately produces relatively rapid results in many KS patients. But he was delayed in raising funds, and so, now nearing the end of his third week in PMH, he was still awaiting treatment. Though medical care, including oncology, is provided as a public good for Botswana's citizens (an African public for whom the term *public health* still has some meaning), as a Zimbabwean national Mr. Makoni was required to pay.

When I arrived in the crowded medical ward with Dr. P, who was meeting this patient for the first time, Mr. Makoni engaged us. He was quite active in explaining his situation. A private, newly diagnosed cancer patient in a public hospital, a Zimbabwean immigrant living in a highly xenophobic time and place, he was desperate.[2] Dr. P looked at me and in that flat tone characteristic of experienced doctors in urgent situations said, "We [meaning Dr. P and myself] will pay for him if need be, but he *will* get chemo this afternoon."* At lunchtime, I headed to the cash machine to get my portion of the money Mr. Makoni would need—no more than the cost of an evening out in New York City—and we phoned the medical ward to request that they send him to us for chemotherapy. An orderly brought Mr. Makoni to oncology in a wheelchair, but when he arrived, he was dead. Mma O, one of the nurses, discovered his passing and called out for Jesus as she pulled a curtain around the cubicle where he sat.

If cholera is what we expect, cancer is not. The countless African cancer patients like Lovemore Makoni have never quite fit into our broader understandings of African health or the community of cancer. In the coming decades this will change, but in the year of Makoni's death, the disease that took his life was just beginning to pierce the collective imagination of the global health and oncology industries.[3] In 1991, in a now infamous memo, Lawrence Summers, then vice president and chief economist of the World Bank, promoted the dumping of toxic waste in Africa because, he suggested, Africans didn't live long enough to care about cancer. He tapped into a long-standing image of African publics as biologically simple ones, an image undergirded by an assumption that infectious disease, fertility, and malnutrition are the problems that matter in African health.[4] Such problems, the reasoning still often goes, are associated with poverty and underdevelopment, while cancer goes hand-in-hand with wealth and industrialization. Summers couldn't imagine

Lovemore Makoni, who at thirty-three could hardly be considered old. Nor could he imagine the fulminating mass on Mary Sedibelo's breast, the blasts packing Boniface Modipane's bone marrow, or the tumor that was strangling Rradikgomo Molefi. Nor could he envision the seemingly endless queue of patients, and the relentless pressures on bed-space in the tiny oncology ward where Mr. Makoni died.

Summers was not alone. Why? How, historically and currently, are Africans envisioned or ignored by the global health and oncology industries, and what impact does this have on the nature of biomedical triage, care, and research on the African continent? If this book examines the PMH oncology ward as a microcosm of twenty-first-century public tertiary care in southern Africa, this chapter shifts scale to consider a political economy of knowledge in Africa, particularly in southern Africa, in relationship to cancer. It traces a history of the alternating invisibility and visibility of African cancers, asking what kinds of biological publics are envisioned in global public health, and what taxonomies of care and prevention ensue from this vision. Such visions are inherently partial: the African political and business elite often travel to European hospitals for their cancer care. Money brings access to metropolitan oncology services, while lack of resources renders the cancers of the broader public invisible to epidemiological attention in contexts where diagnostics are lacking.

In many ways, it seems broader African publics are imagined as people still living in a past where infectious disease and hunger make for a life that is nasty, brutish, and short. There is, of course, a tremendous truth to the hunger and the infections that afflict people.[5] Yet these people are not living in the past. Indeed, their present is an extremely complicated one. The PMH oncology ward and the larger African cancer epidemic subvert the narrow model of infectious disease on which public-health models of epidemiological transition have long been constructed. Indeed, viral cancers are emerging as a profoundly postmodern problem across eastern and southern Africa, one that gains synergy around HIV co-infection. The epidemiological and institutional attention garnered by the presence of these new cancer patients is beginning to unearth a much broader problem of cancer facilitated by shifting ecological (in the broadest sense) and demographic conditions on the continent. Yet the global health community, while beginning to recognize this unfortunate fact, is ill-prepared to respond, given the structures and logics by which they approach Africa. So, too, the metropolitan oncological research community is equally unprepared. Their vast resources — a hybrid of philanthropic muscle, First World government funding, and pharmaceutical company investment — are deployed toward developing new drugs, techniques, and technologies, rather than toward expanding access or tailoring extant therapies and insights to suit African populations in need.

The World Health Organization (WHO) and the International Agency for Research on Cancer (IARC) aptly described this dynamic in 2003.

> Despite many new agents becoming available, often at great cost, the gains in terms of cure rates have been small. Fashion for high dose chemotherapy with bone marrow transplantation, the use of marrow support factors, biological therapies such as monoclonal antibodies or cytokines, have resulted in little overall gain but considerable expense. The driving force for medical oncology comes from the USA, which spends 60% of the world's cancer drug budget but has only 4% of its population [the bulk of the remaining cancer drug budget is accounted for by Japan and Europe]. Huge cultural differences exist in the use of chemotherapy, with USA-trained physicians following aggressive regimens for patients who in other countries would simply be offered palliative care. This has created a tremendous dilemma for those responsible for health care budgets. For example, the use of paclitaxel in patients with metastatic breast cancer will prolong survival by 6 months at a cost of US$12,000. In many countries this would far exceed the total health care consumption throughout a cancer patient's life. Yet the pressure to use expensive patented drugs is enormous. Conferences, travel and educational events sponsored by the drug industry rarely give a real perspective on the effective prioritization of cancer for poorer countries.[6]

As a result, patients like Lovemore Makoni face a situation in which the oncological cutting edge keeps edging up costs and therapeutic intensity with what are sometimes only marginal payoffs for metropolitan patients, while patients in impoverished contexts are often ignored wholesale for lack of funds. In middle-income countries like Botswana patients receive care from clinicians like Dr. P who are buckling under the weight of growing caseloads, while struggling to adapt metropolitan knowledge, technologies, and goods to African biological, technological, institutional, and economic circumstances. In some ways this means practicing a past oncology for contemporary patients, since clinicians must rely only on drugs whose patents have expired and work without the latest laboratory and imaging techniques.[7] In 2010 I watched Dr. V, a Zimbabwean oncologist, hunting through medical journals from the late 1960s. She and her Cuban oncologist colleague at Mpilo Hospital often must go back decades in the published medical literature to debate and determine best-care practices for their patients, even as they strive also to stay current in their knowledge. In the process, the clinical staff, patients, and relatives are left to handle the ethical, intellectual, existential, and personal fallout from this mismatched and imbalanced process of knowledge and technology transfer.

Cancer's African invisibility, its conceptual impossibility, had to be created. Ironically, this has rendered African publics particularly vulnerable to the carcinogenic fallout of global capital. Yet, as we enter the second decade of the twenty-first century, cancer in Africa is beginning to emerge from the shadows through a combination of technoscientific, economic, and epidemiological shifts. The new human papilloma virus (HPV) vaccines, intended to prevent genital cancers, mark new possibilities for recognizing African cancers in an era when private pharmaceutical companies are beginning to pay greater attention to Africa as a site where they simultaneously enact philanthropy and create knowledge and markets. Cancer is made visible once it can fit Africa's extant public-health frameworks, in other words when it is rendered as yet another sexually transmitted disease.

This discussion is schematic. Because of tremendous gaps in our epidemiological knowledge and because of the long gestation period for many cancers, tight etiological arguments are simply not possible for many contexts in Africa. Indeed, this is part of my argument. Cancer's visibility or invisibility in a given population is created through a dense network of knowledge accumulation and production, and this network is uneven or lacking in many parts of Africa. Therefore, this chapter is intended to open discussion of how the invisibility of cancer in Africa facilitates, on the one hand, the production of carcinogenic relationships on the continent and, on the other, clinical knowledge that is often ill-suited to African clinical contexts, furthering the imperative of clinical improvisation. The PMH oncology ward is historically situated within this broader framework of ideas and activity.

Across the globe, understandings of cancer as a "disease of development" does not square with realities on the ground. This should not be surprising. We have long known to be wary of progressive narratives. We know that development trajectories based on specific Western European and North American models do not fit actual economic, political, social, and infrastructural histories from Changsha to Lahore to Bujumbura. Therefore, models of epidemiological transition, which take "development" as their temporal telos, are ill-suited to project or capture the changing burden of disease. Similarly, we know that poverty, racism, and cancer enjoy a troubling synergy, embodied, for example, in the complex production of invisibility surrounding occupational lung cancers for African uranium miners, as described by the historian of science Gabrielle Hecht.[8] Unfortunately, as Lovemore Makoni's experience illustrates, a new dystopic epidemiological narrative is emerging in Africa, one in which cholera and cancer not only coexist, but gain synergy around poverty. This has implications for how we imagine and approach cancer.

INFECTIOUS DISEASE OR THE PRICE OF DEVELOPMENT?

Global public health has long been founded on an assumed developmental telos. The goal has been to mirror the epidemiological transition of Western Europe, Japan, the United States, and Canada. According to this telos, rates of infectious disease, malnutrition, and childbirth would all need to decrease through efforts guided by state and global initiatives, while life expectancy would increase and chronic illnesses would eventually become the significant problem. Most public-health activity in Africa during the course of the past century, animated by a range of competing interests, have developed within this epidemiological progress narrative that has rendered contemporary health in historical terms.[9]

Such narratives have also hinged on a narrow model of infectious disease that has privileged disease transmission over illness. For example, the vast burden of extrapulmonary tuberculosis has long been marginalized from tuberculosis campaigns. Such infections do not facilitate transmission of the tubercule bacillus, but they do produce widespread debility.[10] From the vertical campaigns intended to prevent and halt the spread of infectious diseases, to family-planning campaigns, maternal-child-health initiatives, the primary-care movement of the 1970s, to the fee-for-service health services of the 1980s and 1990s, and the HIV pre-

vention and treatment programs of the twenty-first century, health planners have envisioned biologically simple publics grappling with primary
questions of infectious disease transmission, malnutrition, and fertility.
Statistical collection, which drives health planning and imperatives, accordingly has focused on disease transmission, vaccination coverage,
births, and deaths. And a security framework, sometimes related to
labor-hunger or racialized demographic anxieties, has framed these questions of infectious disease transmission and demography in a politics of
urgency and defense.[11]

Yet if we follow cancer closely, we begin to see a slightly different narrative emerging. Many of Africa's cancers are facilitated by subclinical
infections (hepatitis B, human herpes virus 8, Epstein-Barr virus, human
papillomavirus, etc.) or by chronic clinical infections that over time can
foster cancers. Carcinogenesis is complicated. For example, liver cancers
appear to be precipitated by a combination of subclinical infections with
hepatitis and the presence of aflatoxins in poorly stored African grains.
Human papillomavirus (HPV) facilitates all squamous cell cervical cancers, although many more women have HPV than will ever develop cancer of the cervix.[12] In many cases, however, these disease progressions are
fostered by the immunosuppression brought by malnutrition and HIV.
Well over a decade ago, epidemiologists estimated, "The proportion of
cancers [in 1995] attributed to infectious agents is higher in developing
countries (23%) than in developed countries (9%). This proportion is
greatest among women in Western, Eastern, and Central Africa, where
40% of all cancers are associated with chronic infections."[13] This dynamic may be increasing as more people are put on antiretrovirals, but
it is hardly novel. The recognized relationship between infectious agents
and cancer illnesses is long-standing in Africa.

Half a century ago, researchers in east and central Africa made significant contributions to the field of cancer immunology and to clinical oncology.[14] At the center of this work was a recognition that certain cancers
can arise as co-infections in immunochallenged patients and that silent
(or subclinical) infections matter not only in terms of disease transmission (what I am calling the narrow infectious-disease model), but also in
terms of long-term neoplastic outcomes.[15] In the 1960s and 1970s, when
the bulk of this research was performed, the center of gravity in cancer
research, a growing field, was at least somewhat balanced by the forma-
tion of IARC. Established by the World Health Assembly in 1965, IARC

took up work forged by the International Union Against Cancer, which had included the development of regional subcommittees for Africa, Asia, and Latin America, and which had organized workshops on, among other things, pathologies of particular concern to Africa: Burkitt's lymphoma, primary cancer of the liver, hemangiosarcoma, and so on.[16]

IARC emerged out of a distinct security logic, amid fears that industrial pollutants and other toxins could not be contained within national borders, thus making cancer a key issue for the post–Second World War international community. Initial proposals made this logic explicit, recommending that nations contribute 0.5 percent of their military budgets to form the agency.[17] The agency was founded at a time when "the chemical environment was perceived as the cause of most cancers."[18] At the heart of the IARC mission lay "geographic pathology" or the attempt to compare environments and corresponding cancer epidemiology to determine potential environmental etiologies. This was a paradigm that fostered African cancer research.[19] Environment was understood initially in its broadest sense, to include factors like diet and cigarette smoking, the prevalence of various infectious agents, as well as chemical pollutants, and so on.

And yet, as Nixon declared war on cancer in the United States in the early 1970s and government money flowed into American cancer research, the weight of research and the paradigms underlying its loci would shift decidedly. From 1964 through the 1970s, the National Cancer Institute (NCI) had poured research money into the Special Virus Cancer Program, charged with determining "whether viruses cause human cancer, and if so what to do about it."[20] But the program was later criticized for its lack of results.[21] As Siddhartha Mukerjee explains,

> Cancer biology, the NCI, and the targeted Special Virus Cancer Program had all banked so ardently on the existence of human cancer retroviruses in the early 1970s that when the viruses failed to materialize, it was as if some essential part of their identity or imagination had been amputated. If human cancer retroviruses did not exist, then human cancers must be caused by some other mysterious mechanism. The pendulum, having swung sharply toward an infectious viral cause of cancer, swung just as sharply away.[22]

This process set up an intellectual, political, and economic environment, culminating during the Reagan era, in which molecular biology and genetics began to draw many researchers away from environmental research and into narrower models of inquiry.[23] At the same time, the broader technological field in which oncological research was embedded shifted through the development of new technologies like polymerase chain reaction (PCR) that both facilitated genetic research and put it further out of reach for African laboratories.

There was, however, some limited technological improvement in this period in the form of increased provision of radiotherapy services. Beginning in the 1970s, the International Atomic Energy Agency (IAEA), another agency that would emerge out of a unique Cold War technological context, partnered with the WHO to run programs intended to improve capacity for badly needed therapeutic radiation services in the developing world. The mandate of the IAEA, as an autonomous United Nations (UN) agency, was in part to "seek to accelerate and enlarge the contribution of atomic energy to peace, health, and prosperity throughout the world."[24] Amid the contentiousness of both nuclear power and weaponry, development in the form of healthcare represented at least one rationale that seemed unquestionable. In 1970, sub-Saharan Africa—excluding South Africa, whose services would be racially segregated and profoundly maldistributed under apartheid—had only six high-energy radiotherapy machines. This would increase to twenty by 1989, with technical and training support from the IAEA. Nonetheless, by 1991 the agency could still claim that "only about 35% of the countries in Africa have any facilities for radiation therapy, and in many cases these are grossly ill-equipped and understaffed," a problem IAEA saw as arising at least in part out of the "lack of awareness by the competent authorities of the extent of the cancer problem in many countries owing to an absence of cancer registries and statistics."[25] What was visible to some at the IAEA would unfortunately remain hidden to mainstream oncology for decades to come.

As cancer research moved to the center of metropolitan bioscientific agendas, it was beginning to atrophy in Africa, rather than expand. By the 1980s, with attention being drawn to retroviruses in Africa, the interest in cancer could have gained new import, as some advocated at the time, positing a particularly important relationship and set of research possibilities in the virology–oncology nexus in Africa.[26] Yet war and political predation in Uganda had destroyed the capacity of one of the key oncological research sites in central Africa.[27] Structural-adjustment policies had snuffed out some of the nascent oncology work on the continent, which had showed promise only a decade or two earlier under IARC auspices. At the same time, metropolitan oncological research was coming to emphasize more sophisticated laboratory techniques, genetics, and imaging and drug development, thus widening the gap between African and metropolitan oncology (save for the pocket of metropolitan research in then apartheid-era Johannesburg and Cape Town).

In 1984, in his welcome address to the Symposium on Virus-Associated Cancers in Africa, held in Nairobi and organized by the Organization of African Unity (OAU), the WHO, and IARC, Olufemi Williams, a hematologist and the executive secretary of the OAU's Scientific Technical and Research Commission, described the total lack of African oncological capacity.

> It is perhaps pertinent to stress at this point that there is a severe shortage of trained manpower in the fields of virology and oncology in Africa. It is therefore not surprising that there are very few virologists and oncologists at this meeting. If I were to hazard a guess, I would say that for the whole continent of Africa, which has a population of over 400 million, there is perhaps a ratio of one oncologist to 10 million people and one virologist to 1 million people. These figures may not even be realistic but they reflect the current situation in Africa. In addition to these shortages, there are extremely few institutes of virology or institutes or facilities for cancer research or training in Africa. To quote figures there are less than 10 of these institutes throughout the 50 countries of Africa.[28]

The narrow infectious-disease model of African public health breathed new life through HIV research, and the interest in retroviruses had regained ascendancy but was now decoupled from the complexities of cancer, even as researchers within the United States and other metropolitan contexts began to grapple with the carcinogenic outcomes of HIV.[29] HIV research would offer new insights into immunosuppression that would lead to crucial breakthroughs in scientific knowledge about oncogenic viruses and the viral origins of tumor suppressor gene sequences. Yet this knowledge was not produced with Africa in mind, despite the growing burden of immunosuppression on the continent.

Despite these developments, Africa in the 1990s remained far from the center of gravity in oncology, and oncology far from the center of gravity in Africa. Among cancer researchers, oncogenic viruses continued to be of central concern, and critical work was done at the nexus of HIV- and virus-associated cancers. But without epidemiological support, which proved difficult given the lack of cancer registries and diagnostic and screening abilities, this new work was not sutured to African contexts, where such cancers occur in the greatest proportions. Despite the weight of scientific knowledge, the relationship between viruses and cancers could remain marginalized in the public imagination, as well as in the agendas of global health and development.[30]

One of the reasons for the marginalization of viral cancers was an understanding of cancer as a "disease of civilization." Modern oncology research was founded, in part, on the notion that primitive people living in a "state of nature" exhibited low rates of cancer.[31] This model predominated in Euro-American scientific (and popular) understandings of cancer for the first half of the twentieth century. Africans were long placed outside of history, such that contemporary Africans were viewed by Europeans and Americans as evidencing a static, but deep human past.[32] In other words, American oncology was grounded on a false African twin, such that high rates of cancer in the United States were understood in relationship to the supposed nonexistence of cancers in Africa, creating a set of geographic horizons in American oncology that are only just starting to erode.

If oncology obscured African cancer in the final decades of the twentieth century, African public health, driven in large part by external interests, did likewise, failing to fit cancer into its logics or its politics of triage, despite a promising moment of critical intersection in the 1960s. International health as a domain of professional practice and institutional logic, and as an animating force in the distribution of resources and knowledge, emerged out of a combination of nineteenth- and twentieth-century security concerns brought by global commerce (where ships might unload pathogens as well as goods), and the labor-hunger of European colonialism. This was later furthered by a post–Second World War developmentalist drive to create consumer markets in the global south. Though IARC was conceived in the spirit of international security during a Cold War era of African decolonization, this particular vision of international health proved difficult to sustain.[33] By the 1970s African cancer and IARC itself were rendered outside of the dominant international health vision of Africa with its long-standing focus on infectious pathogens and population control. This marginalization intensified as

[handwritten margin note: cancer was seen as a "modern" disease]

structural adjustment in African public health led by the World Bank and International Monetary Fund (IMF) coincided with the intensive turn to genetics in metropolitan oncology.

PHARMACEUTICALIZED PUBLICS:
HIV AND THE EMERGENCE OF AFRICAN CANCER

The African HIV/AIDS epidemic, which began to be felt in the mid-1980s in central Africa, then spread across southern and east Africa in the ensuing decade, came at a moment when health services in many countries were beginning to crumble in the face of imposed austerity measures and user fees. Across southern Africa, even viable public-health systems in places like Botswana were soon overwhelmed by the huge numbers of gravely ill patients. Many of those patients might have had cancer, but it was HIV that understandably dominated attention. In Botswana, as in other countries in Africa's "AIDS belt," this was a time of existential crisis and widespread loss of life. The public biomedical system offered little to African AIDS patients other than some empirical treatments for opportunistic infections. Little, if any, pain relief was on offer, and more significant, the small but rapidly growing arsenal of effective antiretrovirals developed by multinational pharmaceutical corporations were priced well out of the reach of all but the few Africans who had private wealth or international connections. Africa and its patients were rendered outside of the markets that mattered, and markets had become the mechanism by which healthcare was distributed.[34]

Over the past decade this situation has begun to change, in the face of a new and growing era of public-private partnerships in African healthcare.[35] Markets continue to matter tremendously, but HIV activists have been able to insert moral arguments into the competition between different modes of drug manufacture. Along with political leaders in certain interested and reformist states (like Brazil or India), the activists have succeeded in changing international market structures and controls, producing attendant shifts in the ways pharmaceutical companies approach African patients.[36] Because of these changes, antiretroviral therapies have finally arrived in Africa. In some places, like Botswana, these drugs are donated to an arm of the national healthcare program, which has universal access as its mandate and goal. In others they arrive as part of an uneven patchwork of nongovernmental and state-led services.[37] Either way, this development marks a major moment in what the anthropologist João Biehl has described as the "pharmaceuticalization" of public health.

In this scenario, pharmaceuticals, while incredibly important, are offered in the absence of and as a replacement for hollowed out African health systems. Or they form the nexus for vertical (disease specific) public-health campaigns, which run alongside highly constrained state institutions. Historians might recognize this as a return to the magic bullet campaigns of the 1950s. Meanwhile, as Biehl puts it, "pharmaceutical companies are themselves engaging in biopolitics, gaining legitimacy and presence in both state institutions and individual lives through drugs."[38]

Since the advent of aminopterin over a half century ago, oncology has become a highly pharmaceuticalized endeavor. Yet, given the invisibility of African cancers since the 1970s, and the huge markets in the West for high-cost therapies, which support rapid drug development, places like Botswana would seem to lie outside of the market logics of oncology, even as they have been folded into those of HIV. While this is true to a great extent, the global cancer markets are complex, dynamic, and multifaceted enough to sometimes draw in African patients, rendering their cancers visible.

Most of the drugs in PMH oncology are off-patent drugs developed in the 1970s and 1980s, and manufactured by Indian pharmaceutical firms that specialize in generics. But many newer cancer drugs are still too expensive for use in the ward, even in their generic form. This was the case with imatinib, also known by its brand name Gleevec (or Glivec), which is manufactured by Novartis. Gleevec was approved in the United States by the Food and Drug Administration (FDA) in 2001 and immediately hailed as a wonder drug for patients with chronic myeloid leukemia and gastrointestinal stromal tumors. But it is extremely expensive and must be taken for the rest of the patient's life. In January 2007, during a visit by a team of pharmaceutical representatives, Dr. P asked about imatinib, but the price was well above what he thought acceptable for a public-health system interested in equity. At the time, a standard dose of Gleevec cost well over $3,000 per month for patients in the United States, and even though the price quoted for a generic brand was considerably less, it was still too high given the lifelong financial commitment it would require on behalf of each patient.

However, unlike many other expensive cancer drugs with only marginal benefits, Gleevec, though it could not cure, had also proven re-markably effective, and Dr. P wanted it for his patients. So he began to seek other avenues for acquiring it. After his application stalled with the Novartis office in South Africa, Dr. P approached company executives at a cancer meeting in Europe. With their help, he was able to enroll PMH patients with chronic myeloid leukemia for treatment with Gleevec through a Novartis corporate philanthropy program. This meant sending blood samples to South Africa, where they would be tested for the pres-ence of a specific translocation gene to determine biological eligibility. And it meant collecting personal economic data on each patient to dem-onstrate that they were financially eligible to receive the drug as a gift. By June 2008, a dozen or so eligible patients were called in to PMH to begin taking the drug, which they were told was a gift from friends in Switzer-land.

Batswana patients were not alone in receiving free Gleevec from No-vartis. In 2006 Novartis had already assisted more than "20,000 patients in 80 countries," through its Glivec International Patient Assistance Pro-gram.[39] By giving the drug to those who could not afford it, Novartis was able to fend off competition by the Indian generics industry. This com-petition was not located in southern Africa, as even generic imatinib was too costly for most patients in Botswana. As Stefan Ecks argues, No-vartis's real interest was the markets in the United States and the Euro-pean Union, where they feared that Indian generics could potentially "leak" back in, as could organized patient demand for lower prices. In other words, the global pricing strategy of new cancer drugs like Glee-vec relies in part on gifts to poor patients in the global south, so that a broader community of consumer activism does not emerge to undercut the profits to be made in the global north. At the same time, corporate philanthropy programs in the United States provide Gleevec to Ameri-can patients in need for similar reasons.[40] Drugs as gifts given to some patients sustains drugs as commodities purchased by others, as Eck ex-plains.

The provision of Gleevec for a handful of leukemia patients suggests one small avenue for making African cancers visible in an era of corpo-rate philanthropy. The recent entry of big pharma into the viral oncology market through the development of the new human papillomavirus vac-cines suggests another. Given the synergy between HIV and HPV, and the high prevalence of HPV, African cervical cancer has been rendered visible amid this new, intensively pharmaceuticalized era in global public health.[41] This legibility was accomplished by rewriting cervical cancer through that classic trope in African disease—the sexually transmitted disease (STD).[42]

cervical cancer made visible thru STD

CANCER AS STD: VACCINE IN THE ERA OF THE PUBLIC-PRIVATE PARTNERSHIP

Back in PMH oncology, just across the ward from where Lovemore Makoni's corpse once sat, a row of women with cervical cancer lie in their beds awaiting the van that will take them across town. There they will queue for their turn with the country's only radiotherapy service, a linear accelerator owned by the Gaborone Private Hospital, which serves public patients on the government's dime. Some of these women are actively bleeding, many have serious pain, and all are understandably worried for their futures and those of their children. Each Sunday ambulances from the northern referral hospital in Francistown deposit women with cervical cancer at PMH and the interim home, where patients lacking Gaborone-based relatives may be housed while receiving treatment in the radiation unit. Each week, Dr. P struggles to find beds for these women in this perpetually overcrowded hospital and its satellite dormitory.

On the other side of the hospital, in one of the gynecology clinic rooms, lies the only colposcopy clinic in the southern half of the country. The ministry of health is recommending pap smears for all HIV-positive women, and the clinic has been set up to monitor patients whose smears indicated a high risk for cervical cancer. Here the gynecologist, Dr. T, peers through a special machine (donated by Botswana-USA, or BOTUSA, a partnership between the Centers for Disease Control and Botswana's ministry of health), which has a magnifying lens that highlights the cervix of the woman on the exam table. Peering through the speculum, trying to learn the gynecologist's vision, I am surprised by how clearly a thick, vascular, meaty tumor is framed in the eyepiece. Usually the view is subtler. → *not progressed*

When he finds a suspicious lesion, Dr. T takes a biopsy, making a drawing on the patient's health card to indicate its location. He will use the drawing in a few months, when the patient returns for further internal investigation to confirm and definitively stage the cancer. Dr. T makes these drawings because the hospital doesn't have the glucose solution necessary to see the lesion in the operating theater during the cone biopsy procedure, which is the next step in diagnosis — "They have been ordering it forever,"* he explains — so the drawings guide the clinicians. He says that at home (in central Europe) clinicians cut the cone (a wedge of cervical tissue) and stretch it with pins on a piece of cork so that it doesn't shrink in the formalin, then note where on an imaginary clock (with cervix as circle) the biopsy was taken. Not here, at PMH. Here, he comments wryly, pathology doesn't even recognize that it is a cone.

There is a bottleneck in gyne theater, so the women are booked a few months hence to complete diagnosis and begin treatment. Such patients have already waited six months for the results of their pap smears (given the limited laboratory capacities for processing these tests), then another several months for booking at colposcopy. Many are new to gynecology and have to be taught how to put their feet in the stirrups, and the purpose of the speculum. Some are in too much pain to allow Dr. T a thorough exam. By the time the gynecologist is able to inspect their cervixes and order biopsies, nearly all of those with cancer are too far along for a simple hysterectomy. Many of these patients also have HIV, thus complicating their treatment options and further lowering their chances at cure.

Meanwhile, in a small office at the back of the hospital, near the HIV clinic, Dr. Doreen Ramagola-Masire, a Motswana gynecologist working for the University of Pennsylvania, is piloting a new see-and-treat approach for the country that could potentially obviate the need for pap smears.[43] Dr. Ramagola-Masire examines their cervixes visually, using a solution of either iodine or acetic acid that helps to illuminate any lesions. If she finds a lesion, she removes it immediately. Together with the new HPV vaccines, these see-and-treat technologies are remarkably welcome developments.[44] Though their success depends on well-trained staff, they eliminate the need for the laboratory capacity necessary to process pap smears, as well as the waiting period required for surgery, during which time lesions can progress. So, too, are they garnering a new level of attention to one aspect of the African cancer epidemic.

How well a three-part, high-cost vaccine developed to sell to American consumers will fit Africa's many contexts can only be assessed over time.[45] Not only are there already some concerns as to the long-term efficacy of HPV vaccines in the United States and Western Europe, but preliminary research points to potential problems in African reliance on the importation of technologies developed with metropolitan contexts in mind (as is the case across the spectrum of oncological practice). The two vaccines on the market, Gardasil and Cervarix, address only the two oncogenic (or what are called "high risk") viral subtypes (16 and 18) that are associated with the vast burden of cervical cancer and dysplasia in the United States. Though subtype 16 was the most prevalent in rural Gambia, in some parts of Africa the epidemiology of high-risk viral subtypes for HPV appears to differ from the U.S. context.[46] Evidence from a 2007 study of 150 HIV-infected women in urban Zambia, for example, found that high-risk HPV strains 52 and 58 were more common than HPV 16 or 18 in women with high-grade squamous intraepithelial lesions or squamous cell carcinoma. Within Africa and beyond, "studies are unanimous, thus far, in showing that HIV-infected women are more commonly infected with non-16 and -18 high-risk (HR) HPV types, such as 52 and 58."[47] Moreover, aggregate data suggests that 50 percent of HIV-positive women in sub-Saharan Africa who had HPV 16 or 18 were co-infected with another HPV type.[48] But data are still inconclusive about the extent to which "non-HPV-16 and -18 types persist in actual CIN3/cancer histological specimens of HIV-infected women."[49] Even where a vaccine targeting 16 and 18 is biologically appropriate, questions remain as to whether the suppression of prevalent oncogenic viral subtypes (in this case, HPV 16 and 18) through vaccination might provide an opportunity for selective pressure by other, currently less prevalent oncogenic subtypes within a given population. Furthermore, in the United States these vaccines were tested for their suppression of precancerous cervical lesions, but far less is known about how effective they are in suppressing cancers themselves in a context where precancerous lesions are rarely detected and, in particular, where HPV and HIV are locked in a deadly synergy.[50] One reason the bioscientific community understands relatively little about the complexities of HPV in Africa, despite the high rates of genital cancers, is that such knowledge ultimately hinges on the combined presence of population-based cancer registries, with accurate clinical data, and sophisticated laboratory ability to test for HPV within cervical cancer specimens or in women who are suffering them.[51] Yet such infrastructure is lacking in the very places where cervical cancer poses its greatest threat.

The rewriting of cervical cancer as an STD fits one element of cancer into the old epidemiological narrative of African public health without interruption. And, not surprisingly, the new HPV technologies fit neatly into the evolving logics of public-private partnership that are restructuring global public health. Merck pharmaceutical, developer of Gardasil and partner in Botswana's pioneering national ARV program, has committed to donate $500 million worth of the vaccine (valued at the price it commands on the U.S. private market) to programs in twenty-three "of the world's poorest nations."[52] This move is a first step toward establishing this new and still controversial vaccine into the basic vaccination schedule in the developing world.

Genital cancers matter tremendously in human terms in places like Botswana, where countless women are suffering and dying from cancers of the cervix and vulva, so these vaccines are awaited with cautious optimism. And Merck has proven a generous and important partner in Botswana. Perhaps it is necessary to render a cancer as an STD for it to make sense within the logics of African public health, yet the reduction of complex pathology to vaccine-preventable STD threatens to erase cancer's complexity through an infectious disease versus chronic illness schematic. Indeed, synthetic estrogens, tobacco, and other toxins appear to combine with HPV in facilitating genital cancers. And the high infection and death rates from cervical cancer in Africa are as much about the lack of comprehensive women's health services (such as those Dr. Ramagola-Masire is attempting to develop for Botswana) as they are the sexual networks that the STD logic and the HIV co-infections imply. In other words, the STD logic, the narrow infectious-disease model, points toward pharmaceuticalized and behavioral interventions. Meanwhile, the cancers themselves point toward the need for more broadly conceptualized forms of care. Nonetheless, viral cancers, now entangled with HIV, STDs, and the pharmaceuticalization of public health are regaining visibility as an extended form of infectious disease.

CARCINOGENIC INVISIBILITY

In 1996 I joined staff from the local clinic at a village meeting in eastern Botswana. Such meetings are common in the country, where a history of participatory democracy and public communication have meant that meetings—between a family group, a neighborhood, a village, or an age cohort—have been central to political and social life since long before colonialism. Colonial and postcolonial bureaucratic and development initiatives eventually co-opted the meetings as a standard form of communication. This particular meeting was well attended although it took place in a relatively minor village, because the paramount chief of the *morafe* (the sub-ethnic polity of the area) came. I have attended many public meetings in Botswana, but I remember this one in particular because of my surprise when the chief stood up and began lecturing about *motsoke* (tobacco). My Setswana wasn't good enough to follow everything he said, but I understood clearly when he lit a cigarette, blew the smoke through a piece of white cloth, then held the cloth up to show the nasty brown stain the smoke had left behind to everyone gathered. At a time when such meetings often included demonstrations about condoms and lectures about tuberculosis, the chief was talking tobacco.

Many of the men listening to the chief that day were former miners, as were many of the men lying in PMH oncology, quietly hungering for breath under their oxygen masks, or awaiting their next meal of Ensure through the nasogastric tube taped to their nose and threaded via the surgeon's knife through the narrow opening in an esophagus now crowded with tumor. For much of the twentieth century, the majority of able-bodied Batswana men from the southeastern region of the country crossed the border to work deep underground in South Africa's mines.[53] The system of oscillating migration, where African men left their families to live in mine compounds for extended periods of time, only returning home for short visits, became a defining feature of southern African history. From as far away as Angola and Malawi, and as close as Lesotho, Botswana, and Mozambique, able-bodied men disappeared into the bowels of South Africa, Southern Rhodesia, Swaziland, and South West Africa to bring forth gold, asbestos, diamonds, platinum, uranium, and other minerals. The profits were channeled along transnational, institutionally racist lines. The southern African system of colonial migration was pathological, creating a perfect delivery system for the dissemination of malnutrition and tuberculosis, then, later, HIV (and HPV).[54] It drew men into gold mines where radon daughters emanated from the rock.[55] It produced mine waste laden with asbestos and uranium-laced tailings. It also created new markets for commodities like commercially manufactured cigarettes and alcohol, and new modes of consumption. It created cancer while depending on its invisibility.

If rendering genital cancers as STDs has helped them gain scientific *mining industry exposure*

visibility and funds in southern Africa, the same cannot be said for rendering esophageal or lung cancers as occupational risks associated with the complex ecology of the southern African mining industry. There are several reasons for this. In this region, with its high rates of endemic tuberculosis and overstretched public-health and diagnostic infrastructure, lung cancers are routinely misdiagnosed as tuberculosis (TB) and treated with antibiotics. Indeed, many of the PMH lung cancer patients underwent TB treatment before they were referred to Dr. P, who finally established a proper diagnosis. It is impossible to know how many more such patients die without access to a proper diagnosis. Moreover, tuberculosis appears to increase lung cancer risk, so there is the possibility of a plural diagnostic need.[56] Occupational and environmental health hazards associated with industry are often difficult to establish. Multifactoral models of causation based on occupational or environmental exposure are complex to establish and made all the more challenging by the long gestation period for cancers. Industry commands resources, including access to data, and therefore can produce doubt about causation through preemptive science, whereas workers and community members are often ill-positioned to seek research that serves their interests.[57] Historically, these dynamics were exacerbated in southern Africa, where until recently African workers and community members were systematically denied legal and political rights.[58] In other words, the scientific and epidemiological invisibility of radiation and asbestos exposure and their effects on miners were structured by racial-capitalist logics that have historically made occupational health a key concern in the region.[59]

Despite the fact that Africans produce 26 percent of the world's uranium, Gabrielle Hecht demonstrates that occupational radiation exposure in places like Namibia became invisible through intertwined global scientific and geopolitical erasures of African nuclear activity.[60] In South Africa, for example, the Witwatersrand gold mines are rich in uranium ore. Surveys of radon exposure in the mines performed in the mid-1950s found relatively low levels, and autopsy data failed to reveal excess rates of lung cancer among miners. South African scientists thus concluded that "high ventilation standards" in these gold mines and "stringent safety precautions" prevented occupational health hazards. Yet, as Hecht explains, this science, like subsequent studies undertaken in 1971 by the South African Atomic Energy Board (AEB) in collaboration with the Chamber of Mines, masked the political economy of race.

These studies were done at the height of apartheid. Race structured exposure. The AEB study, like those in the 1950s and 1960s, were based on average radiation levels taken in only 10 percent of the mines. White miners worked shorter shifts, and were positioned in the cooler, intake airways, where ventilation cleared the radon. Black miners worked the rock face, where the radon built up at much higher rates, in some places "reaching ten times ICRP [International Commision on Radiological Protection] dose limits."[61] Yet the South African scientists based their claims on autopsy data taken from exclusively white patients. They dismissed the exposure of black patients by claiming they were temporary migrants; yet most miners, like those coming from places like Botswana, would cycle through the mines to accumulate decades of work.

The scattered asbestos dumps that stretch across northern South Africa to Botswana's southern border also bear this history of the invisibility of exposure, skewed science, and the cultivated invisibility of cancer.[62] For much of the twentieth century, South Africa was a leading producer of asbestos. The raw material was sent to the global market, while the tailings "were used extensively in building materials and road surfaces in former mining regions."[63] Children played on mine dumps and in some cases attended schools built from asbestos-laden brick. Tailings and sludge wound up in drinking water. As the pathologist and historian of science Lundy Braun has established, the carcinogenic effects of all this asbestos, and the political and economic logics that structured hazardous exposures, were part of an "invisible epidemic" of asbestosis and cancer. One doesn't need to travel to West Africa where "tonnes of toxic waste from British municipal dumps is being sent illegally to Africa," nor to Somalia's Puntland coast, where, as both United Nations officials and Somali pirates have reported, Asian and European toxic and nuclear waste has washed ashore, to see the problem of carcinogenic waste is not limited to Lawrence Summers's failed World Bank proposal.[64]

Toxic waste isn't the only carcinogenic market relying on the invisibility of African cancer. Africa is now a target market for the tobacco industry in flight from shrinking U.S. and Western European markets. General Agreement on Tariffs and Trade (GATT) and, later, World Trade Organization agreements opened new possibilities for transnational distribution of cheaper tobacco in the 1980s and 1990s.[65] As with toxic waste, successful activism in the West (resulting in stricter domestic regulations and successful litigation) has inadvertently exported carcinogenesis to

Africa. Unlike in Asia, where tobacco use has recently escalated alarmingly as tobacco corporations open vast new markets, the African "cigarette epidemic" is in its early stages in many parts of the continent.[66] In other parts of the continent, most notably South Africa, cigarette consumption has declined from its peak in 1990. This is at least in part the result of a significant public-health campaign, including new laws which since 2000 have limited smoking in public places.

Data is partial. Figures on tobacco consumption are lacking for many places on the African continent. This is part of the difficulty in ascertaining the extent to which tobacco may or may not be a growing problem. According to the World Health Organization's *Tobacco Atlas 2002*, high figures for smoking in Africa include an estimated 65 percent of men and 35 percent of women in Namibia; 66.8 percent of men and 31.9 percent of women in Kenya; and 59.5 percent of men and 43.8 percent of women in Guinea.[67] I have been unable to corroborate these extremely high figures against other sources. But, given the targeting of African nations by tobacco multinationals, which have been gradually buying up local plants and scaling up advertising efforts, and given the rapidly increasing rates of total cigarette consumption on the continent, there appears to be an upward trend under way in at least some places on the continent.[68] It will be decades before the cancerous outcomes of all these cigarettes become apparent, yet the prospect is frightening in places like Botswana, Namibia, and South Africa, which already have some of the highest rates of esophageal cancer in the world.

In 1994, as Americans entered the era of intensive, successful anti-tobacco litigation, Annie Sasco, an epidemiologist at IARC, sounded the alarm in a column in the pages of *Tobacco Control*. Sasco made an appeal for basic epidemiological data that was sadly lacking. Her plea underscored the ignorance of African cancer evident in the field of development economics only a few years previously, in Summers's World Bank memo. Sasco cited estimates that cancer mortality data only existed "for about 9% of the population, and cancer incidence for 0.5%."[69] Even as epidemiologists, social scientists, and bench scientists poured into Africa to produce knowledge about AIDS, multinational tobacco was taking advantage of the production of scientific ignorance around cancer in Africa.

As the historian Allan Brandt puts it, "The industry's assertion that harms deemed unacceptable in the affluent West are tolerated in the developing world smacks of a dubious moral calculus. It implies that people in India or Egypt really don't object to dying of cancer so long as they were spared from TB or cholera. Common sense suggests the fundamental flaw in this logic."[70] And of course, this same logic is the one that underlies the transfer of toxic waste — or even a World Bank economic plan for the same. Yet as cancer becomes highly visible in Africa, such logics fall apart. The family of Mokwena Mosiepele, a sixty-eight-year-old man (perhaps a former miner) who lay dying with metastatic lung cancer in PMH oncology in February 2007, found his condition tragic. Did it matter to the late Lovemore Makoni that he died of cancer rather than of tuberculosis? We will never know.

Africans are living in a carcinogenic time and place — and this fact is producing much misery and loss. Yet their cancers and the carcinogenic relationships that underpin them remain mostly obscured, due to the progressive developmental model that has long guided African public health, regardless of biological and social complexities on the ground. This model facilitates carcinogenesis, even as it marginalizes the needs of the hundreds of thousands of African cancer patients.

THREE

Creating and Embedding
Cancer in Botswana's
Oncology Ward

To what extent is cancer in Gaborone the same thing as cancer in New York City? What happens when a known biomedical object like a tumor appears in new contexts as part of an emergent epidemic? How is that object then constituted in different political-economic, sociocultural, technical, and biological circumstances? How do patients come to learn the nature of cancer in contexts where oncology is only just being established? These are what some scholars would call ontological questions. They are not abstract, but rather carry tremendous implications for care.

Historians and philosophers of science and medicine use the term *ontology* to explain how scientific objects, things like germs or gamma rays or DNA, become recognizable as distinct entities. It takes an array of technological, intellectual, social, political, and economic circumstances to perceive these entities and make them widely accepted as facts. Cancer is no different; it has a history. In fact, it has more than one. Cancer in Botswana and cancer in New York City have come into existence, are experienced, and are defined through particular technological fields. They are created or made sense of through particular social, cultural, and historical categories of meaning. These histories overlap, but not entirely.

For example, in one sense pre– or early-stage breast cancers (BRCA1 and BRCA2 genetic markers, ductal carcinoma in situ, and lobular carcinoma in situ) do not exist in Botswana. They may be biological processes taking place inside some women's bodies, but this fact is not part of the clinical or personal experience of the disease. For women in Botswana and their clinicians, breast cancers are palpable, symptomatic things. In North America the rise of screening technologies and mass screening efforts mean that such precancers and early cancers are regularly discovered in women's bodies, and have engendered vigorous ethical, political, and policy debates.[1] Screening itself arises out of a particular constellation of philanthropy, technology, medicine, and feminist politics, among other forces. These early and pre–breast cancers have important effects. They propel women into surgery and more intensified forms of surveillance. Women imagine that invisible cancers might be growing in their breasts and they are rightly fearful of such possibilities.

In Botswana by contrast, pre– and early breast cancers cannot be perceived by available diagnostic tools.[2] They are generally not part of public or clinical discussion around breast cancer, nor of how women regularly imagine breast cancer or the possibilities held within their own bodies. On the other hand, massive, fulminating, necrotic breasts, breasts that have essentially been auto-amputated by aggressive late-stage cancers, used to exist in the United States, but are now incredibly rare because mass screening and awareness (which helps produce the "precancers") means that most women receive care before their disease has progressed to such a distressing state. Not so in Botswana, where over 50 percent of women who arrive at PMH with breast cancer are inoperable, though attempts are made to downsize the tumors with chemotherapy in hopes of making mastectomy possible. Many of these surgeries are what are called "toilet mastectomies," meant to rid the patient of a breast now profoundly disfigured by a necrotic, suppurating, and stinking mass. In PMH toilet mastectomies are far more common than lumpectomies. These are issues of disease ontology.[3] In the early twenty-first century, breast cancer in Botswana and breast cancer in the United States have a great deal in common with one another, but they are not exactly the same thing.[4]

In addition, a woman in North America with breast cancer will experience her disease at least partially in relationship to a set of expectations around what breast cancer is and what treatment might entail, further crystallizing some boundary around this disease. This is not to say that she will understand the disease in the same biomedical terms as her doctor. When I asked a class of about forty, very smart, American, advanced undergraduate students what a tumor was, only one could offer a basic, plausible definition, though several had close family members who had suffered from cancer. For an American woman, breast cancer will be a profound learning process, but even this fact is something she will have reason to anticipate. She will most likely know other women who have had breast cancer, she will see fundraising appeals, she might join a support group. She will come to her cancer with at least some vocabulary—of symbols (like pink ribbons), words (like *chemotherapy*), and images (like hair loss)—that will help her make sense of a very challenging therapeutic pipeline. She will most likely know that a biopsy or a CT scan are diagnostic practices, while irradiation or a chemotherapeutic injection are therapeutic ones.

In Botswana, while there have long been cases of breast cancer, in the absence of oncology they did not spawn a collective experience or image of the disease and its attendant biomedical processes among Batswana. As a result, lay expectations around the disease are still extremely thin, as is the vocabulary of symbols, words, and images. Over the past decade, cancer-prevention posters have started appearing in government hospitals, but many of them are produced by a small NGO, the Cancer Association of Botswana, which appears to reproduce metropolitan posters with messages that do not resonate in Botswana, because the images are too foreign or because they presume a very different health system.[5] Articles occasionally appear in the local newspapers about cancer, and there are occasional radio or television segments. Depending on her educational level, a newly diagnosed breast cancer patient might look on the Internet to find more information. But for most patients this vocabulary and set of expectations, this sense of what cancer is, will develop in large part through her own illness experience. A breast cancer patient in Botswana will learn through her own experience that a biopsy or CT scan is diagnostic, while irradiation or a chemo injection is therapeutic. Let me be clear. It is not that biomedicine is unfamiliar in Botswana. If cancer is an empty category only just now filling up, HIV, hypertension, diabetes, and tuberculosis are well known or even overdetermined. So our patient with breast cancer will also learn to separate her cancer from her hypertension or her HIV. This too is part of ontology or disease creation, as individual patients establish the nature of their affliction.

To pursue these issues and their implications for patients and their caregivers, I examine the ontology of cancer in Botswana during an emerging epidemic. I trace how phenomenological experiences of pain, palpation, bodily change, fear, nausea, and, often, rot merge with techno-

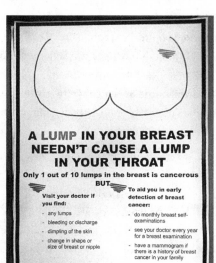

Breast cancer awareness poster suggesting that women who suspect breast cancer
get a mammogram—but mammography is not publicly accessible.

scientific practices of cytology, chemotherapy, radiation, and surgery to
create cancer in PMH oncology, and how clinical communication reveals
the highly unstable nature of this new entity. I focus, in particular, on the
interactions between patients and the oncologist in an effort to understand the microprocesses by which this cancer epidemic emerges on the
clinical ground. This is temporal work. Patients arrive in Botswana's oncology ward and clinic often after months or even years of seeking diagnosis, often with late-stage cancers, and with great anxieties about their
bodies and their futures, anxieties shared by the clinical staff. Dr. P and
his patients often find themselves envisioning different futures and managing different horizons of hope, which over time merge into a gradual
if often unsatisfactory alignment through the processes of treatment. I
pay careful attention to how somatic experiences, clinical communication, and treatment modalities combine to create and manage futures
for patients whose knowledge of their disease is built bodily as well as
cognitively.

*I ask Michael how his prostate cancer began, and he tells me it started with
pain and itching in his eye. Now he is facing the prospect of an orchiectomy.*

Dr. P asks Rra Tladi whether his esophageal cancer is better or worse after two rounds of chemo, and Rra Tladi complains of shoulder pain. Dr. P says, "No! That does not matter. Is this"—he points to the swelling in Rra Tladi's neck—"bigger or smaller than when you started?" "The same." "Can you swallow porridge?" "Yes." "Well, then it is better—when you first came here you couldn't even take mageu [a soft porridge]—so the treatment is working—we continue."

Such examples from my field notes begin to reveal something about cancer in Botswana. We see the political economy of hormone-therapy pricing making orchiectomy (the surgical removal of the testes) the only affordable treatment for advanced prostate cancers. We see that patients do not necessarily sort their symptoms based on some already established baseline knowledge of cancer or biomedical physiology. Thus esophageal cancer can manifest itself in painful shoulders and prostate cancer can begin with painful eyes. We see an oncologist managing large numbers of patients, with skeletal medical records and limited imaging services, attempt to gauge therapeutic efficacy through brief clinical interactions by getting patients to focus on the mass.

This oncology ward or these patient experiences are not so radically different from a ward in an undifferentiated imagined "West." Certainly, there is a political economy in New York City (where I live) that determines treatment options, wait times, and outcomes. Memorial Sloan-Kettering (a leading cancer center) and Kings County Hospital (a large public hospital) share the same major metropole, yet a quick comparison of the two challenges the notion of unity in experiences of oncology in New York City. And it is not only in Botswana that patients mention troubling symptoms that doctors find irrelevant to the condition at hand in their attempts to gauge the efficacy of a particular treatment. But in a country, like Botswana, with universal access to care in a health system initially designed to grapple with infectious disease and maternal-child health, where patients do not have a primary-care physician or internist with whom they have an ongoing relationship, where the only cancer ward is in a public hospital, where cancer is newly emergent and trailing behind a profound AIDS epidemic, and where biomedicine is far from hegemonic, such details begin to sharpen our sense of how cancer is enacted here. We see it crystallize through brief clinical encounters in which patients learn to localize the phenomenology of pain in a mass, through chemo-induced vomiting in a hospital where the most powerful anti-emetics (like Kytril) are too costly to use in any but the most extreme circumstances, and through brutal if hopeful practices, like amputation, in a system where less alarming alternatives are sometimes lacking.

CREATION AND REFUSAL

Bringing cancer into being isn't easy in Botswana, and it is often quite painful. But, since 2001, it has been done every day—sometimes partially, often imperfectly—by a lone oncologist, a rotating staff of medical officers (residents), a shifting team of nurses, and a bevy of patients and their accompanying relatives in PMH, a hospital that lacks a cytology lab, an MRI machine, endoscopy, and mammography, where histology is a dicey prospect, tumor markers unavailable, genetic screening impossible, and patient counseling ad hoc and fleeting if it occurs at all.

Cancer is made biomedically intelligible in partnership with patients for whom the experience of their cancers is often quite pressing. Because Botswana generally lacks prevention and early detection programs for cancer (though a cervical cancer screening program has begun), many patients are diagnosed only when their disease is advanced. Since cancer is also emerging amid a profound AIDS epidemic, it is often occurring in patients whose existential angst and hopes are also shaped by an HIV diagnosis, as is their experience of biomedicine under a newly pharmaceuticalized regime.[6] And co-infection with HIV renders cancers more aggressive and prognoses more ominous and uncertain, and necessitates adjustments to standard treatment regimens.

Many try to deny cancer an opportunity to root in their bodies. "I already have AIDS, I cannot now have cancer too. I will just wind up frustrating myself."* So a woman with HIV told a Congolese doctor as she refused his recommended pap smear during her regular meeting with him at a primary hospital in the Kalahari, where she had come to collect her ARVs and check on her progress. This woman was not alone. Many others are refusing cancer. In most cases, of course, it cannot be put off forever. The phenomenological urgency of cancer overwhelms even the most fearful or stubborn, and thus begins the crystallization of debility—of pressing pain, disfiguring growths, and the stink of rotting tissue—into something called cancer, a something that will be built in layers and enacted through routinized pain, nausea, needles, wound care, ultrasound jelly, and submission to the rhythms of a small oncology ward in an overcrowded hospital.

Though most of my attention in this chapter is on patient-doctor interaction, I hasten to underscore that this phenomenology (or bodily consciousness) is socialized in contexts well beyond the clinic door. At home, relatives wake in the night, worrying over and attempting to massage away the severe pain of loved ones. Patients dizzy and nauseous from chemotherapy lean on their sisters or mothers for support during numerous trips to latrines in family yards. These same sisters, mothers, and daughters help clean necrotic cancer wounds at home (or they don't), and come to the ward in the evenings to bathe their patient (or they don't). Young men and women accompany their aged grandparents to the clinic for relief. Some usher patients with deeply stinking tumors into the oncology clinic for care when the smell interrupts their ability to eat and socialize at home.

Mosadi, age thirty-four, finally confided in her sister-in-law that she was worried about her breast. A hard mass in it had been growing for two years. When her sister-in-law saw the profoundly deformed breast, which had a massive tumor about to break the skin, she was seriously alarmed and brought Mosadi straight to PMH oncology. In another instance, a mother, herself a cancer patient, dragged her twenty-three-year-old son into the clinic by the ear and ordered him to pull down his trousers for the oncologist. "Look at what he has been hiding!" she barked, a single fat tear rolling down her cheek as her son stood silently exposed next to the exam table. That morning she had accidentally caught a glimpse of his legs, which he had been striving to conceal — his thighs were severely swollen, thick, and riddled with KS lesions.

It is not only patients who might initially attempt to refuse or forestall cancer. Nurses and doctors, too, in clinics and primary hospitals across the country, routinely deny the oncological suffering of patients — until finally cancer is diagnosed at PMH (though this is beginning to change). There is something familiar in these stories. In the United States as well, many people (especially women, whose worries and pains are more easily dismissed) tell stories of doctors who missed their cancers until it was too late. Others have avoided medical institutions because they fear the costs or because they lack citizenship and fear the state. In Botswana, however, this dynamic is furthered by a health system in which the ability to recognize cancer is highly concentrated, localized in one place: PMH

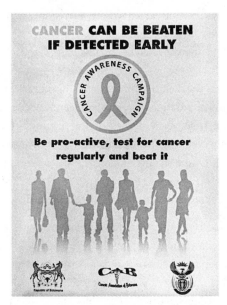

Cancer screening poster.

oncology. Patients cannot directly access PMH oncology in search of a diagnosis. They must be referred by a doctor at a primary or provincial hospital, or by another specialist within PMH (whom, again, they could not have accessed without referral).[7]

Doctors who staff the primary hospitals and nurses who staff the clinics have had almost no training in cancer.[8] A nurse in a local clinic told Sekgabo, a mother of four who was in her mid-thirties at the time, that the painful, hard lesions on her face were the result of the bad things she had been putting on her skin (the implication being that she was using skin lighteners). On another visit, her laborious breathing was attributed to possible TB infection, and she was put on TB treatment. After several such visits, her gums and upper palate having become extremely painful, she finally bypassed her clinic and local primary hospital, and made her way to the dental clinic at PMH, where Dr. O, the maxillofacial surgeon, immediately suspecting Kaposi's sarcoma, referred her for HIV testing and sent her to Dr. P for a consult. By the time she arrived in oncology to confirm her cancer diagnosis and begin chemotherapy, the cancer was in her lungs, covering her legs, destroying the lymphatic system, and causing massive swelling in her knee. Her pain was intense—as was her disfigurement. Two years later her KS was in remission, but her left knee had become a fixed joint, so she could walk only short distances, she had lost her job as a cashier, and she lived in chronic pain. Cancer is nothing if not insistent.

Cancer emerges for these patients as a disjuncture between bodily experience and clinical practice — a gap that eventually closes through the dispensing of pain relief, the (often temporary) shrinking of tumors, and the discomforts of therapy. Mma Bontle, a sixty-five-year-old woman, explained to me how she struggled to establish her cancer, until finally it crystallized into the nausea of chemotherapy and the existential angst of serious illness. Her story of delayed diagnosis is an all-too-familiar one.[9]

It is almost two years now since this problem started. I was going to the clinic, and the clinic referred me to the provincial hospital, to the doctor that does problems of the head and face. So at that time the problem was that I was losing my voice, and also that the ears were always itching, and I wasn't really comfortable with that itching, like deep inside, and I didn't know what was happening. So then the doctor there did some evaluation, and she found that when she opened the mouth, in the throat there were some flesh there that were, like, growing too closely. The gap was closing, and also at the time I was having lots of nose blockage. So she took some samples of what was in there to see what it is, and then from there I was told to come and get the results. When I got there, the doctor said, "Ah! I couldn't find anything, but I will try to liaise with other doctors," to help me.

So I continued with this hospital, but they couldn't find anything. Then at some stage they had to cut some piece from there and then send it to South Africa for more investigations, but still they couldn't find anything. And then I was referred to PMH, to the ENT [ear, nose, and throat specialist], who gave me Panado [a mild analgesic], of which I had to ask for it, otherwise they wouldn't be giving me anything. [At that time, PMH did not have a formally trained ENT, just a medical officer assigned to that post — and a set of instruments.]

It was even getting worse, getting swollen, and the glands, they were getting swollen, and the ears. So I went back to the provincial hospital. When I got there, the doctor also wanted to cut — that would be the third time, so I complained, "*Wena*, you can't be cutting, cutting all the time. I came here complaining of my ears, and now you are cutting and cutting somewhere else, and you are not replacing. And now I have this wound, which I don't know what it is." But then at last I agreed. They took another piece. I went, and when I came back, they gave me the results. Whilst waiting for the results, I heard over the radio, there was some information of cancer. They were talking about how cancer develops, and they mentioned the glands being swollen, and so I thought, "Ao! Can this mean that I am having cancer?" But I didn't say anything. I just kept that information.

When I went for the results, the doctor said, "I couldn't find anything." She wanted to cut—to cut for the fourth time. There now I said, "No, this time you are not going to make it. If you are fixing an old car, you get out the old part, you put in a new one! But for me you are not fixing anything, only taking parts out! Not replacing." This time NO, I refused. *Ke a gana tota! Ke bua nnete.* [I truly refused! I am speaking the truth.]

At this point, my friend Dikeledi, who accompanied me at the interview, and I burst out laughing. Mma Bontle joined us, amused all over again by her own cleverness with that white lady doctor.

So I refused that day, and then I said, "I came here without a wound and now I have a wound. If you can try to heal this wound, then I will be happy—otherwise there is nothing you are going to take from me again." So then the doctor said, "OK, I am referring you to PMH." So the doctor phoned while I was there, because I was just sitting there without anything being done. So the doctor phoned and wrote a letter, and then off I went. So from there, when I arrived at PMH, I met Dr. P, who actually promised to help me, and he said he is going to take some fluids from those glands—it actually injected and then it was taken, it was very painful when he took it. *Botlhoko! Yooooooo! Yoooooo! Ke a tshaba!* [Pain! Ow! Ow! I am afraid!]

So I was told to come for the results the following day. When I arrived early that morning, I was there, seated outside in the queue, when Dr. P saw me and pulled me into the room. And then I was told now that it's cancer. And then I was, like, scared and didn't know what to do. I don't know exactly what I was scared of, but I was scared. And then I was given the bed. And on admission I was put on the drips—which were making me sick. I was vomiting.

So I have put everything onto God. If I die, I will be dying for God. If I get better, still I will be living for God. I wasn't told what cancer is—but

I didn't bother to ask what it is. All I knew was that I had cancer and the doctors were going to help me.

VERNACULAR ONCOLOGY

Patients travel many different routes to arrive at PMH oncology. They share one common experience though. On arrival they will be seen by Dr. P, who will then winnow through and triangulate their usually terse explanations of bodily experience with knowledge he creates through multisited practices (i.e., palpation, cytology, ultrasound). Though he does little prognosticating with patients, except to threaten them with death if they refuse treatment, he will imagine a future trajectory for them in ways they yet cannot, and he may chastise them for coming "late" for treatment when the disease is already advanced and their fates more or less sealed.

Dr. P arrived at PMH from Zimbabwe in 2001. The halcyon days when work in Zimbabwe appealed to an idealistic German oncologist were long behind him. In PMH he works hard, and he works seven days a week.[10] He handles all outpatient clinical oncology, seeing usually between twenty and thirty patients a day (though the worst days bring up to forty patients to the clinic), directs a twenty-bed ward (where capacity is overstretched and extra beds are often packed in), and supervises aspects of care for cancer patients housed in other wards in the hospital. He is also the hospital hematologist. He feels the contours of lumps, lymph nodes, tumors, skin, and organs on the patient's body. He smells necroses, listens to whistling lungs and gurgling tracheostomies, and lays his hand on the back of each patient during ward rounds to feel for fevers. The nurses joke about his thermometer-like "magic hand." He performs fine-needle aspirations, extracting cellular material from lymph nodes and possible tumors, pressing it onto slides. He also aspirates bone marrow and performs bone-marrow biopsies by boring into the sternum or pelvis of a patient and extracting a core sample to slice, or a tube of blood and fragments, to place on slides. Since the hospital lacks a cytology lab, he is also the one to examine the slides under the microscope, actively blocking out his image of the patient's clinical presentation as he places a drop of oil on the slide, then searches for tumor cells. Cytology, as he told me, "is like trying to understand the architecture of the house from a few bricks."* But he strives to make cytologically based diagnoses

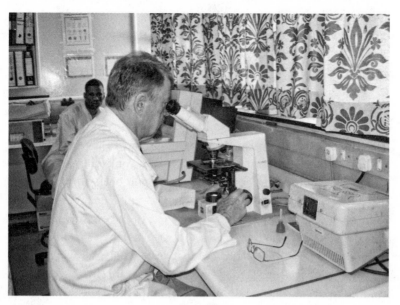

Dr. P, the cytologist.

and to avoid requesting biopsies, because waiting times for minor theater are long, as is the wait for histological results, which can take weeks. He also tries to avoid the need for histological confirmation because there are numerous errors and inconsistencies in the reporting of histology. Indeed, one of the pathologists appeared to be unable to adapt to the rise in cancers he was now asked to diagnose (fortunately, he is no longer on staff), and so ordering histology was something of a gambling exercise. If a biopsy was read by the competent pathologist, it was enlightening; when read by the incompetent pathologist, a biopsy might well be useless or, worse, dangerously misleading.

Though there are two experienced radiologists on staff, who Dr. P regularly consults when their greater precision is needed, the demand for imaging studies at PMH is tremendous. So where possible Dr. P also performs ultrasounds (on a very old ultrasound machine he rescued from the trash and rehabilitated) and reads X-rays, searching for enlarged spleens, echo-rich bright spots in kidneys, the white circles of bone metastases, and other images that help him create physiological processes out of patient symptoms. Nurses at PMH do not insert cannulas (needles which are attached to the intravenous tubing or to a syringe) except in emergencies, so the oncologist also dons gloves, ties tourniquets, and inserts needles to administer the tubes of chemotherapy, sometimes helping patients to the sink to vomit after a push injection of cisplatin.

It was the responsibility of the ward medical officer to administer chemotherapy, and Dr. P would assist with the final patients in the queue when he finished his clinic for the day. Yet some of the medical officers were so burned out from the grueling nature of their work that they would sometimes fail to show up for work, arrive late, or call in sick. Others were dedicated but had to grapple with competing responsibilities. In 2006, and for much of 2007, there was only one medical officer in the ward, Dr. A, who was hardworking and extremely smart but also had night and weekend duties in the medical wards, and eventually in anesthesiology. And he also went on leave, to visit his family and to seek out opportunities for further training so that he could specialize in anesthesiology. During this time Dr. E, a Cuban primary-care physician, was also assigned to oncology, but she severely injured her leg and spent several months out sick. Furthermore, Dr. E did not like working in oncology, which was far from her area of expertise, so even after she was mobile she often stayed in the medical wards or found reason to leave early. She also made repeated errors inserting cannulas, which made her loathe to administer the chemo. (Inserting a cannula to administer chemotherapy is a critical task, even if it is a routine one. If the needle is not firmly in the vein, then the chemo drugs can leak into the flesh. Since the drugs are cytotoxic, they destroy the flesh and are released into the tissue, where they are taken up by adjoining cells in a continuing process that is dangerous and which produces extremely painful wounds of raw open flesh.) As a result, there were many days and even weeks when Dr. P took care of the entire ward, all of the outpatients, and then administered the chemotherapy.

Dr. P writes the sick-leave forms for patients and the guarantee forms for the ministry of health, which pays for citizens to take radiotherapy at the private hospital across town and occasionally to receive certain sophisticated treatments at a private oncology practice in South Africa, and he signs the death certificates. He pushes against the bureaucracy, striding in and out of the pharmacy, demanding the chemotherapy, asking the pharmacist to search for necessary supplies or drugs as they go out of stock, delivering patients personally to radiology or surgical consults so that they are not set aside or delayed. He counsels the families of patients, sometimes "popping money out" of his own pocket, as they say in Botswana, to buy a meal or otherwise assist a destitute patient or familial caregiver in need of material help. He teaches the visiting ethnographer to read the slides with a teaching microscope. He is interviewed each year on the radio during Cancer Awareness Week. He funds the annual ward Christmas party. In 2009 I spent twenty minutes helping him devise a temporary clamp for the broken chair he was regluing in the clinic office.

This oncologist continually tacks back and forth between different kinds of firsthand knowledge, creating cancer and the cancer patient in multiple registers simultaneously (visually, tactilely, socially, microscopically, clinically, economically, bureaucratically), rather than in a series of disconnected or abstracted parts, as is the case in a larger oncology setting, with a more complex division of labor.[11] But what is this cancer that he labors to birth? When I began this work, in 2006, cancer in Botswana was a novel entity in all senses. There had long been cancers in Botswana, but they were not united in a popular lexicon under a unified diagnostic rubric.[12]

And so the oncologist's diagnostic pronouncement might be the first time the patient or her relatives have ever heard the word *cancer* (or its Setswana cognate: *kankere*). Some days I would marvel at patients who burst into tears on learning that they did *not* have cancer, but TB instead. Tuberculosis was feared, and perhaps shameful—cancer, by comparison, had been their hope. Or perhaps the patient had heard a story on the radio, like Mma Bontle had, or had seen a poster in the clinic or hospital, or had heard of a friend or neighbor with this disease, which happened increasingly. Then the person might know to be scared, without knowing much else. Between 2006 and 2009, this changed amid a rapidly escalating cancer epidemic. Many Batswana came to fear cancer, which was now recognized to be a powerful disease, though little else was known about its contours.

For the oncologist, too, cancer as it emerges in Botswana today is somewhat unique. Each month *The Lancet Oncology* arrived in Dr. P's office. His shelves contained four of the same core medical reference books I have seen in oncology offices at the Dana Farber Cancer Institute in Boston. And in 2009 I lugged eighteen pounds of brand-new oncology reference books to Gaborone for Dr. P, who tries to ensure the ward has the latest editions. He attends at least one international cancer meeting a year. Cisplatin is cisplatin, and 5-FU is 5-FU, after all.[13] Dr. P uses a creatinine calculator he picked up from a pharmaceutical rep in Germany; he stages tumors based on international standards. Yet what he encounters each day renders this knowledge ever so slightly tenuous.

Cancer in Botswana differs from cancer in the global north, where it lies at the heart of cutting-edge, highly capitalized biotechnical research, and of public narratives about loss, heroism, and hope. Botswana is so far on the periphery of the oncological imagination that its biological, epidemiological, sociocultural, and technical context is beyond the conception, much less the concern or evidentiary basis, of most oncological research, with its emphasis on new drugs, expensive screening technologies, molecular and genetic knowledge and interventions, and costly procedures such as bone-marrow transplantation.[14] Fewer studies address the challenges of simultaneous HIV and tubercular co-infections in treating cancer.[15] Yet because of drug interactions and compounded side-effects, and because some of Botswana's cancer patients are too immunocompromised to withstand standard chemotherapeutic regimens, charting a treatment course for patients who are co-infected with HIV and cancer is difficult.[16] Newer "smart" drugs like herceptin are too expensive to consider, and important support interventions like neupogen, for treating the neutropenia that is a common side-effect of chemotherapy, are too costly to use in any but the most compelling of circumstances, though Gleevec is available for some patients through a corporate philanthropy program. And nursing conditions are also different in PMH, such that the support care necessary to enable, for example, concurrent radiotherapy and chemotherapy (the standard of care for many cancers) is not possible. Evidenced-based oncology protocols published in the leading medical journals do not address what to do when etoposide, 5-FU, or cisplatin—all core chemotherapy drugs in PMH's stripped-down arsenal—suddenly go out of stock, as each did for some time in 2007. Thus, in order to envision the possible futures of Botswana's cancer patients, their oncologist must borrow, adjust, and even deny, but never simply import metropolitan knowledge.

Because he is working in a context where the biological, technological, and institutional circumstances are both unstable and somewhat different from the norms on which clinical research is based, Dr. P must not only fully understand the published literature, but also be able to work empirically. In other words, he often must chart a treatment path that is based on evidence and experience. This form of reasoning is an integral part of oncology everywhere, as doctors must make decisions about specific patients, often in the context of competing scientific claims and probabilities. There are moments in the trajectories of cancer illnesses or survivorship when therapy becomes an "experimental zone in which innovation and guesswork is dominant."[17] In the United States such reasoning is further complicated by the specifics of various insurance schemes that determine therapeutic possibilities for any given patient. In Botswana, the uneven infrastructure and mismatch between local biological and institutional circumstances and the context of the published research amplify the need for these intellectual moves. Here are a few moments from my field notes on an unremarkable June day in 2008 which underscore the necessarily empirical nature of Dr. P's work.

> As we search for blasts in a bone marrow slide, Dr. P tells me, "In leukemia you can only measure true remission through PCR—but here I can only do it with a bone marrow slide—you say remission when there are very few blasts, not more than 5 percent in the marrow slide."
>
> Because of the overcrowding at the radiotherapy machine, they are giving higher doses per day, so the number of days is shorter. "This is not a good idea," Dr. P says.
>
> Dexamethasone has been out of stock for months. Morphine is out of stock, substitute codeine.
>
> There is a man in Male A bed 2 with Hodgkin's who is HIV-negative, emaciated. He wants to be checked for TB. Dr. P says, "He is smart—we should not be fooled, even though Hodgkin's is a wasting disease." TB and Hodgkin's have a synergy—Dr. P has found both in the same lymph node.
>
> We see the woman with non-Hodgkin's lymphoma. She is better, but still very sick. She will continue with etoposide. We have seen the foamy vacuoles in the malignant cells [lymphoblasts] on the slide from her aspirate—Burkitt's. She has one eye that is sunken and doesn't move, which indicates central nervous system involvement, and so will get a lumbar puncture this evening. Dr. P says that the standard of care in the West for Burkitt's with CNS involvement would be to begin with radiation to the brain. "But here we cannot do that because we don't have the support care necessary, and because patients with HIV make it less possible. The protocols have pushed up the cure rate to 60–70 percent, but we can't do it with HIV patients—we would kill the patient."

Then a team comes from pharmacy—around 3:45 PM—[but] they don't have the chemo. The hood in pharmacy has been broken for weeks.[18] *The British company that made it is trying to milk the government out of an exorbitant rate for repairs, despite the fact that the machine is less than two years old. The pharmacist went to the Institute for Health Sciences [IHS, the nursing school] next door, and the lab with the hood they have been borrowing was already locked for the day. Dr. P starts yelling, "So now you want to expose us to the cytotoxic drugs. You need to mix them, and you need to make arrangements with those people at IHS [and ensure] that they cannot leave early without communicating. You are trying to shirk your work and make us do it!" The nurse agrees. They want us to be the ones exposed. The pharmacist tries to defend himself: "Tell the patients to come back tomorrow." "No! These patients have been waiting all day, they cannot come back tomorrow for treatment. They need it today!" Then Dr. P yells again and says, "No, fine, I will mix the drugs." He is furious. Then he and the medical officers start mixing, and joking about cytotoxicity. Drs. P and H and M reminisce about how for the first few years after the ward opened in 2001, they used to mix all the chemo here on the open table without a hood. So they mix the chemo, and Dr. P puts in the cannulas. This, too, is dangerous work—the majority of the needles will have HIV on them, and eventually many doctors will get a needle stick in the chaotic crush of work [as happened to Dr. R, Dr. E, and Dr. A during my time in oncology]. Hospital nurses do not insert IVs except in the case of emergencies. It is in their contract.*

As we sit searching the slides for tumor cells in the quiet hum of the lab, Dr. P remarks, "Normally you should see at least four slides but I am lazy today." It is 6:45 and work began eleven hours earlier, so I do understand why he is only looking at two or three slides per patient. He's right, this is actually work best done first thing in the morning, when you are clearheaded and with fresh eyes, but that is difficult here. When he finally gets home, after his dinner, he will then turn to the day's paperwork, which is extensive.*

The cancer that Dr. P is making into a biomedical object shares space with tuberculosis and HIV. It is a fuzzy sort of cancer, one that is hard to bring into the kind of sharp focus that PCR, MRI, mammography, colonoscopy, and other such technologies enable. It is fuzzy, too, because Dr. P's work involves a tremendous amount of "unbracketing," to use the philosopher Annemarie Mol's term.[19] In other words, though he is in part working empirically, relying on evidence from the patient and experience from the previous cases he has treated, he cannot take the evidence before him for granted. Instead, he must think about how the information is produced, then decide if it is reliable. If his cytological diagnosis does not fit with the clinical picture, he might revisit the slides, wondering if he was too tired the night before, when he read them. If the patient's physical appearance and reported symptoms do not match the results on the pathology report, he must then ask himself if the report is reliable and strategize a way to corroborate or overturn it.

His work is artisanal and empirical, yet he must also rely on others: medical officers work under his direction in the ward; basic blood tests are done at the laboratory by technicians; surgeons must be consulted about potential biopsies, dilations, and amputations; gynecologists refer patients with gynecological cancers; the pharmacists dispense drugs for outpatients and often mix the chemotherapy; the pathologists at the national laboratory perform histology; nurses and nursing assistants translate between Setswana and English; nurses clean necrotic wounds, assess patient condition, take vital signs, and dispense treatment; and each day Dr. P must consult with the two radiation oncologists from the private hospital across town, where public patients are sent through a public-private partnership.

In this process of collaboration, too, Dr. P improvises. For some time, he had been locked in tension with one of the PMH surgical specialists, Dr. F, who did not share Dr. P's sense of urgency and therapeutic imperative. Dr. F developed the habit of not hearing his pager in the drowsy hours after lunch, which he took at home, when he saw it was oncology on the line. In response, Dr. P began paging Dr. F from Accident and Emergency, knowing Dr. F would think it a surgical emergency. Dr. F returned the calls, but soon began to refuse to return to hospital grounds when it was Dr. P who summoned him. Over time, Dr. P developed ever more elaborate ruses to trap Dr. F. I recall the look of defeat and irritation on Dr. F's face one balmy afternoon in April 2007, when he arrived in Accident and Emergency only to find a triumphant Dr. P standing waiting for him. After a pregnant pause, and to my profound amusement, one of the medical officers exclaimed, "Checkmate!"

As Dr. P repeatedly stressed to me, and as is evidenced in his daily clinical routine, it would be a grave mistake at PMH to bracket the messiness of practice and the practicalities of measurement. Was the patient really hypertensive or were the new automated blood-pressure cuffs not working? Was the tumor really inoperable, or was the notoriously lazy surgeon simply seeking to shirk his work? Was this really a hepatoma, or was the pathologist wrong? Was the patient really anemic, with her tongue so pink, or did the lab make a mistake? In an African hospital (even a relatively well-funded one like PMH), with its ill-maintained and often second-rate or donated equipment, expired drugs, unpredictable supply chains, and with many disaffected and a few grossly underqualified staff (among the many other excellent and committed staff, I hasten to add), one must lead with unbracketing.

CONSOLIDATION, TRANSLATION

Dr. P was too busy to create *all* the knowledge himself, and too ignorant of and distant from the fullness of patient lives to fashion all the different aspects of cancer and the cancer patient, so he had to learn when and where to cultivate trust. He was not alone. Patients, too, had to learn who to trust in a bureaucratic and overwrought health system, already bruised and dulled by the pains of a long AIDS epidemic. Trust in this case meant accepting, at least provisionally, that cancer was indeed the problem and that relief would be forthcoming. Many patients had already sought help from Tswana or Christian prophetic healers, to no avail. Others were among the many Batswana who refused Tswana medicine on intellectual or moral grounds, or who simply could not afford it.[20] Any of these pathways made them more open to biomedicine, even if they were not interested in its logics. In a few instances, after newly diagnosed patients offered me polite but stunned looks in response to my attempts to explain cancer in biomedical terms, a nurse might say, "This doctor is very good. He is going to help you." Or Dr. P might say, "You will hate my treatment, but it will help you." Such patients often looked immensely grateful for these pithy declarations. That they had arrived at a legitimate site of help, of care, was the first, most crucial piece of knowledge that many of them sought. In other words, tenuous yet hopeful trust was often born in moments of desperation or of relief at finally having come to the end of the diagnostic pipeline.

At the same time, the move from diagnosis to the rigors of oncology — which might involve amputations, chemotherapy, nasogastric tubes, colostomies, tracheostomies, and other such distressing prospects—was a sudden and in some ways totalizing one.[21] In order to enact this move, knowledge production and disease creation (ontological emergence) need to be brought together to consolidate cancer.

13 June 2008

I have been asking the nurses and nursing assistants [who also do a substantial amount of translating between patients and doctors] "How can you explain lymphoma in Setswana?"

Mma S says, "It is VERY difficult—you can't do it, you have to explain it in relation to a mass—sometimes using kgeleswa *[abscess]."*

Mma R [recently transferred from female orthopedic ward] says, "Nna [Me], I am new here. I don't know the diseases yet."

Yesterday I asked E [one of the nursing assistants]. He says, "No, translation here is a very big problem. I don't like to do it." And then, "Nna, I don't know what is this lymphoma." I then try to explain to E that it is in the system in the body that carries metsi *[water] and dirt in channels through the body—but I am not sure that clarifies.*

Dr. S says it is like a colander you use when cooking to catch all the small stones and dirt when you are rinsing food. I think this is a good analogy and will try to remember it.

For any oncology ward to partner with patients and their relatives in the refashioning of pressing bodily experience *as* cancer, doctors and nurses must communicate complicated and frequently jargon-laden biotechnological truths into accessible language, often resorting to analogy. Where translation across languages is also at issue, as it often is in Botswana, matters are further complicated, as some objects and processes expressed and understood in English simply cannot be rendered in Setswana. Biomedicine has become *the* therapeutic system of global health programs—its practices rely on purportedly universal bodies, technologies, and things. Proponents of biomedicine like Dr. P understand the objects of biomedical practice to be materially obvious. Yet the challenges of clinical translation in a place like Botswana reveal instead the instability of medicine's objects.[22] This instability shapes the communication and action that form care for desperately ill people in a place where biomedicine is expanding enormously and becoming more and more technologized.

Linguistic translation is recognized as critical in biomedicine. At the very least, doctors need access to patient experience through communication, and patients need to understand doctors' instructions in order to comply with treatment guidelines. For Dr. P, who must constantly bracket other forms of knowledge, translation is crucial in determining the efficacy of any given treatment. Is the mass shrinking? Does the patient have pain in places that suggest bone metastases and require X-rays? And of course, proper communication is necessary for patients and their relatives to make informed decisions about therapeutic options.

That translation is linguistic is not surprising. But translation is also critical in the ontological sense—it is a necessary, foundational means by which the nature of cancer is created in Botswana. Over time, translation brings new entities into being, then embeds them in the bodies and environments of patients. These new entities are not neutral—they have a politics that is endowed through translation. One of the clearest examples of this ontological genesis through translation can be seen through the creation of the CD4 cells in the wake of the antiretroviral rollout in Botswana, beginning in 2002.

In Botswana as in many parts of Africa, the human body is understood and inhabited in slightly different ways than we find in contemporary biomedicine or metropolitan lives. For example, organs begin and end in different places or combine together in different systems, and there are different relationships between people or between human and non-human actors, be they ancestral shades or bacteria that engender illness or sustain health. In the late 1990s, when the AIDS epidemic picked up pace, saturating the public landscape with imported health messages (including radio, newspaper, billboards, public meetings, and didactic community theater) and through ubiquitous clinical encounters in HIV clinics, testing facilities, hospital, and primary-care sites, one saw a few translated entities crystallize and previously nonexistent entities come into being. The same biomedical machine continued its long-standing and unsuccessful attempts to erase, extinguish, or marginalize other long-standing Tswana medical entities like *sejeso* (poisons associated with witchcraft), ancestors, or divination bones.

HIV itself was rendered as *mogare* (the worm), building on fifty years of history in which bacteria, viruses, and parasites had merged into a single translated category, one that enjoyed an awkward coexistence with other Tswana entities of dirt and pollution. Finally, its boundaries sealed off, mogare began to swim through the social body, and the bodies of the sick and the well. Mogare had become *the virus*! More significant for the ontological politics I am trying to describe, a whole new, robustly signified entity was created and embedded in the human body through ubiquitous practices and powerful domains of translation.

When I worked as a participant-observer in home-based and clinic care in Botswana in the 1990s, there was no Setswana term for the immune system. It was a concept that was skirted around and never directly tackled. Across a range of therapeutic systems it was agreed that some foods, for example, were body building and body protective, but underlying ideas as to why were left unmarked. Beginning in 2002, however, as the government began to implement the first national antiretroviral program in Africa, a new kind of immune system crystallized around the CD4 counts now routinely performed and discussed as a necessary part of the ARV program. But in the process, the CD4 count, as a proxy for the immune system as a whole, was translated into Setswana as *masole* (soldiers). Thus Batswana now envision themselves as internally armed with regiments of soldiers, the size of their inner army being a proxy for how healthy and strong or weak and vulnerable they are. The drugs they take promise to increase or stabilize the number of soldiers in their individual army.[23]

Similar processes of translation are under way in North America, for example, even if we look only at how medical knowledge is produced and disseminated among English speakers. There is nothing obvious about having an "immune system," and its ontological history originates in early-modern European legal concepts and international relations, as Ed Cohen's work has elucidated.[24] But if we look at how this plays out in a place like Botswana, where biomedical knowledge is not hegemonic but rather part of a more metaphysical world, we see ontological emergence and the basic pragmatism of clinical communication combining in a political and economic context where the possibilities and moments of translation are fleeting because patient queues are long and time with the doctor is short.

In PMH oncology, facilitating cancer's ontological emergence through fleeting moments of translation was very difficult indeed. Unlike in the HIV clinics, which operated through a didactic structure, wherein patients were drilled on their disease knowledge and expected to perform rituals of biomedical compliance, PMH oncology was working

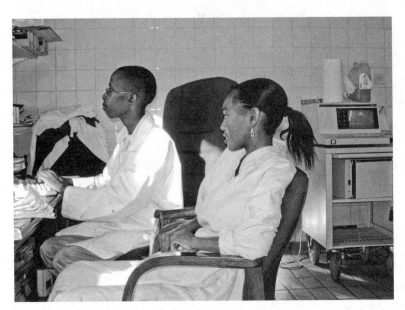

Translating in the clinic.

ad hoc. There were no professional counselors in oncology (unlike in the field of HIV, where the new paraprofessional job of HIV counselor was pursued by many Africans as one of the few new emergent routes to employment). And Dr. P was far too busy, impatient, and directive to initiate lengthy discussions with patients about the nature of their disease. The nurses, for their part, tried to fill in the gaps, but they were also quite busy, and except for the ward matron and a new nurse who arrived in May 2009, none of the nurses had training in oncology.

Initial diagnostic conversations were usually quite brief, and would go something like, "You have kankere. We will now treat you with injections. This injection might make you vomit, it might make you lose your hair, it might make you dizzy. This is temporary. Your hair will grow back. You must come for six injections. First today, then three weeks later, then three weeks, three weeks, three weeks, until we reach six injections. When you come for injection, come early in the morning. Get your blood drawn at the lab, bring the lab result here, and then take a number and join the queue. Do you understand?" Or, for a new inpatient, "You have cancer of the mouth. We will give you a bed and shrink it with medicine."

Kankere is the Setswana word for cancer (a cognate term). But beyond that, to what bodily processes does it refer? Such details emerged only over time and through repeat visits, as patients learned to ask questions and began to separate diagnostic from therapeutic procedures, as brief conversations aggregated into meaningful knowledge. In March 2007, a seventy-eight-year-old woman who had previously been treated for cancer of the colon was surprised that Dr. P aspirated a lymph node in her neck when her pain was in her lower abdomen. She asked me why he did that, and I explained that there are *ditshika* (veins, channels, nerves) that connect the abdominal organs and the *leruo* (swelling). So he can take metsi (water, fluid) from the swelling to check if the disease has planted seeds elsewhere, or if this is a new disease. *Wa bona?* (You see?) *Ke a utlwa.* (I understand.)

April 2009

Tlotlo, the woman who wears the brown Dutch print two-piece, with KS on her legs, comes in. She completed radiotherapy in October. She had six courses of chemo in 2005 and four in 2006. The wounds are mostly dry, but it looks like a little bit of KS is coming up. She is having hot flashes, weakness, tiredness, and palpitations. I try to present the issues to Dr. P. He asks about her period. "It is skipping some months and then coming every day." "Where did they irradiate?" "The pelvis was in the radiation field." Dr. P says, when I interject to tell him her response, "It is not my job to tell you about this—I am not an expert in irradiation—but it could be menopause. You should ask those people [the radiation oncologists at GPH, the private hospital where the radiation is administered] to explain to you what is happening."

As he goes to do something else, she and I talk, and I explain about early menopause, ovaries, and popelo (womb), and she says, "OK, I understand." I look concerned and ask, "Do you have any children?" "Yes, two—I am not worried about that, I am only worried about my health. I don't need any more kids," she says matter-of-factly. She asks, "So chemo and radiation can do that?" I say, "Not chemo, only radiation." She says, "OK, I see, you know all my friends from the radiotherapy, when we went together to GPH, we are all having this problem." I ask [where she talks to them]—and she doesn't necessarily talk to them much at home—but she saw them on the bench outside just now, and they were chatting. When she leans forward, I can see that this woman who speaks excellent English is also wearing waist strings from a healing church.

There was supposed to be a nurse or nursing assistant present to translate between the German oncologist Dr. P (who spoke English) and the patients and their relatives, many of whom could not speak English. Much to my discomfort, however, when the nurses were busy with other tasks, it sometimes fell to me, with my highly imperfect knowledge of Setswana, to translate. Even when a nurse was present, translation often turned into a team effort, as we struggled to render cancer — with its cells, platelets, lymphatic system, metastases, tumors, radiation, and so on — into Setswana language and regimes of embodiment. With Dr. P frustrated and rushing us, we tried to seal off patients in their own envelope of skin (so their relatives wouldn't think them somehow toxic and segregate them), and to rhetorically create and inject cells, tumors, and metastases into the individuated bodies of the patients, often using agricultural metaphors (seeds, roots, weeds) or biological analogies (sores and meat). We made an incinerator out of the linear accelerator, and the medicine of white people out of the chemotherapy, careful to avoid the Setswana word for poison, *sejeso*, given its implications of witchcraft and purposeful harm.

Knowledge of cancer emerged piecemeal, with new bits being translated over successive clinical encounters, and with patients discussing their situations with one another during endless days spent lying in the ward or during the lengthy hours they spent on the benches awaiting treatment or clinical time. Even before these fragile entities were precariously in place — or so we hoped — patients were expected to commit to the doctor's treatment strategy. The etiquette of the clinical encounter in Botswana, an outgrowth of colonial, missionary, and mine medicine, has long been based on a top-down model. Patients do not expect to ask many questions. Yet, while some patients were content to leave expert knowledge to the doctor, many others expressed a pent-up desire for biomedical knowledge, knowledge that might give more precise shape to their existential and phenomenological concerns. Some sought information on the Internet. Mma M, the ward matron, was wonderfully adept at answering questions and offering explanations, a task she tried hard to make time for, but she was also extremely busy running the ward.

As someone who had more time to spend in conversation than did the clinical staff, I could clearly see the desire for knowledge as I conducted interviews with cancer patients. Although the interviews were intended to further my own research into their lives and perspectives, patients would often turn the tables and begin to question me. They sought detailed explanations of side-effects, the logic of treatment decisions, and possible prognoses. I gradually gained a reputation as someone who would at least try to answer such questions, and I found myself appreciated for this service. Many patients told me that my explanations often confirmed knowledge gained elsewhere (which was reassuring to me), but also added an analytic perspective, which sometimes revealed to them some new aspect of the underlying logic of oncology.

The lack of robust knowledge and explanation on the ward was, not surprisingly, a problem for some patients. Rra M, one of the nurses, explained it well.

> When a patient doesn't know what to expect and why they are doing this, often they might end up defaulting, and then we yell at them that they are irresponsible! Even when I go to translate into Setswana, there are not words, and with each patient I am trying to match my knowledge with theirs to figure out how to say it, to gauge what they know. Even when I say, "No, you can't have treatment today because your blood is down," — well, this is hard to explain. "No, not blood pressure — I mean these pieces inside of the blood. . . ." [And the patient says,] "What do you mean, I have pieces in my blood!!?" Wa bona? [You see?]

Importantly, not only did Dr. P's words need to be translated for the patient, but the reverse was true. Dr. P cannot speak Setswana, nor can he always understand the vernacular forms of embodiment effaced by translated speech, or the terminology and reference points through which patients conveyed their critical concerns.

26 June 2008

A man with acute lymphocytic leukemia; he is sixty years old. Dr. P uses the occasion of this patient to do some teaching. He brings the medical officers in and gives them a big lecture about leukemia in which he basically says the prognosis is bad. He is speaking in English, assuming this old man cannot understand, and he never directly addresses the patient during this speech. Then the medical officers leave, and the man sits down and says to Rra M, the nurse (and the only Motswana in the room), "No, I am brave, and even though they say I am dying, I will face it. Let the lion come to my house. I will not shrink." Dr. P asks for the translation, and Rra M gives it. Dr. P mis-

understands this seane *[proverb] and says, "No, you cannot just give in and*
say let the lion come." So I say, "No, he is saying the opposite. He is daring
the lion—'Let it come, I am not afraid. I will not give up easily. I will fight.'"
Dr. P is impressed with this man.

CYCLICAL TIME, EMBODIED KNOWLEDGE

Based on clinical conversation alone, fewer patients, no doubt, would
submit themselves to oncological treatment. But the cancers being made
into specific biomedical objects in Botswana are rarely asymptomatic.
More often they are built out of large, hard growths, blocked throats, debilitating edema, infected necrotic wounds, and troubling pains. Patients
bring the fullness of bodily experience and affliction to their cancer trajectories. From there, the oncology team works to hone and localize the
cancer into a biomedical object, and most important, to "blast away" or
"destroy" the cancer which is plaguing the patient. It is really around the
promise of healing that cancer is consolidated in Botswana. Yet healing,
for all its urgency and potentially beneficial ends, is not pleasant work.

In the clinic office, newly instantiated cancer patients begin to learn
their own form of vernacular oncology. Treatment becomes another
pipeline, one that is often cyclical, as patients come for rounds of chemotherapy and clinical follow-up. In the process, an oncological habitus of
sorts is built, deepening the phenomenology of cancer. Cervical cancer
patients, who I watched struggle with the novelty of the exam table in
the colposcopy room or while receiving a pap smear during their time
in the diagnostic pipeline, soon learn to climb on tables, put their feet in
the stirrups, and bare their genitals for pelvic exams as a matter of course.
Men with esophageal cancers remove their tracheal tubes, clean, and re-
place them without flinching. Patients hold their arms out and pump
their fists for blood taking and chemo injections. Those awaiting chemotherapy with "anticipatory nausea" developed through previous experience learn to sit where they cannot see or smell the chemo room. Others
have learned to crave rather than fear the painful puncture that will bring
relief when a swollen knee destroyed by KS or a fluid-filled pleural space
is drained. And, of course, many socialize their changing bodies through
laughter—as when Mosadi arrived for her third round of chemo, removed her hat to reveal her newly bald head, turned to Mma D and me

with a wink and a nod, and drove us into scandalized laughter by saying, "But the hair loss is all over [my body]. I am young again!"

Patients might wait for several hours or even all day for their turn in the chemo room, bored and anxious about how they will manage the bus journey (and then walk) home. They chat with one another (and their accompanying relatives) on the bench, trading information, and encouraging and commiserating with one another, or they sit silently. They spread out a cloth and sleep in the cement breezeway outside the ward. They complain loudly at anyone who tries to jump the queue. But despite their desire to make their way to the front of the queue and then return home, entering the chemo (or "treatment") room is a thoroughly loaded experience.

In the treatment room the woman with the mastectomy and the lump we are watching finishes her injection. The old man with lung cancer lies on the table getting his one-hour drip. She is in the chair. She is finished, but looks green and doesn't stand up to go. Dr. A says she looks nauseous. I take her to sit next to the sink to wait. Then I give her some damp paper towels to hold, and wipe her forehead with another. After a minute she says, "OK, I can wait outside." She rejoins the bench, and the other patients ask after her. She just says one word: sebete *[liver, nausea]. I call the next patient in—the lovely and chic woman with breast cancer. She is wearing a dark, wool pantsuit and a beautiful wig with bangs. "My God,"* she says, and then in Setswana, "Modimo o ntusa"* [God help me], and braces herself to enter the room.*

She cringes as the cannula is put in; it is painful. It has to be replaced from the crook of the left arm to the right hand, because it infiltrated on the first vial. Immediately after it is all in she goes to the sink and vomits, as I am ripping the tape for her arm. I put it on the gauze as she vomits, and then I get her paper towels. She washes her mouth, collects herself, and leaves.

The kind of learning I've just described underscores the stakes here. These are patients with a very serious and often tremendously painful disease who are now undergoing challenging therapies, therapies that might call for disfiguring surgery, deeply nauseating medicines, scorching radiation burns, severe mucositis, and countless minor insults, therapies that often render young women infertile. In Botswana, where nearly a quarter of the adult population is HIV-positive, and where everyone has intimate knowledge of AIDS and its suffering, it is telling that HIV was

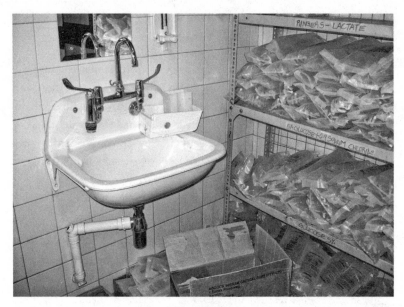

The sink in the chemo room.

the benchmark patients used as they struggled to convey their experience of cancer. "If only I just had AIDS," was the ironic refrain I heard repeated many times by PMH cancer patients.

Oncology requires a kind of totalizing commitment. Part of instantiating cancer is creating its urgency. Most patients cannot work, at least during the first week after receiving a round of chemotherapy, which is usually administered every three weeks. Many spend from several days to more than a week with overwhelming nausea and vomiting after they return home from their chemo treatment. Those who receive radiation face several weeks or months without work, during which time they must grapple with burns, sores, and other side-effects. Patients who are regularly employed are entitled to paid sick leave, but those who make their living through casual labor, domestic service, petty trade, and agriculture must manage the economic consequences, as must those patients whose employers cheat them out of sick pay. Each appointment means countless hours spent waiting in queues for a turn with the phlebotomist, X-ray technician, oncologist, or surgeon. Patients must also be prepared with money for transportation to and from PMH, which may entail expensive bus and combi fares.

Those whose cancers require three- or five-day inpatient chemo treatments or other hospitalizations must surrender themselves to the ward totally. In May 2009 Rra P lay attached to a chemo drip in the ward and received a call on his cell phone informing him that his younger brother had just died. Despite his grief, and his considerable responsibilities as eldest brother in making important family arrangements at this critical time, he was not allowed to leave the hospital earlier than expected. He needed to finish his chemo course and the postchemo hydration IV; only then, three days later, could he return to his home village, which was several hours away by bus, and begin the mourning process. And, of course, amputations—whether of cancerous breasts, penises, legs, feet, or testicles—entail lengthy periods of hospitalization and debility.

Cancer does not wait. Part of disciplining patients as biomedical subjects means creating temporal urgency. Sometimes this points backward, perversely rationalizing a bleak future. Clinical staff, especially Dr. P, chastise patients for having "delayed" in seeking treatment or for "running away" from treatment, thereby earning the label of defaulter. But these are radically different envisioned pasts. Many cancer patients look for the origins of their disease in episodes of trauma: a breast cancer brought on by a blow to the breast, perhaps by an abusive husband; cervical cancer as an outgrowth of genital sores first brought on by witchcraft in childhood. Others experienced biomedical refusal at Botswana's clinics and primary hospitals, where genital cancers are often mistaken for STDs, leukemias for bouts of flu.

Amid all this, because of all this, efficacy too takes on a compounded urgency. It needs to be established as the nexus on which all this communication and activity founders. And efficacy, in this setting, is far narrower than patients might initially hope. For Dr. P, efficacy means shrinking a tumor, and preventing or halting the process of metastatic spread. For patients, efficacy means feeling better and enacting a socially and physically meaningful future. It means seeing one's children safely to adulthood. Bridging these two horizons of hope necessitates a further consolidation of cancer as a biomedical object, one meant to be separate from and foreign to the patient's self. If patients with solid tumors can be persuaded to focus on the mass, different horizons of efficacy held by the patient and the clinician can be partially merged, and patient hopes reinvested in biotechnological modalities.

But cancer is not a stable entity; its phenomenology is porous. After cancer is established, perhaps in only skeletal and shadowy form, it continually threatens to overspill its delicate etiological boundaries. And so patients come with shrunken tumors, but suffering from infections and other complications. Dr. P attempted to marginalize such complaints, shoring up the boundaries of cancer, even as he treated the side-effects of disease or therapies where possible. "Yes, yes, but that doesn't matter. Is *this*"—pointing to the tumor—"smaller or larger than when we started?" he would say to someone who had come in miserable from an infection but with a shrunken tumor, even as he wrote the order for the necessary antibiotics on the patient's card. When patient misery was iatrogenic, Dr. P usually shared a thin laugh with the patient over the absurdity of their predicament, even as he sought to recalibrate hope by peeling cancer (as relevant somatic experiences and symptoms) off the fullness of the body. So, too, the nurses might diffuse the violence of therapy by rendering it absurd.

> The tumor is packing the esophagus, and Dr. R fails to put in the NG tube. So Dr. P supervises the next attempt. Afterward, Mma S does a HILARIOUS imitation of him putting in a central line with force: "You must PUSH, PUSH!" She imitates him with a Bic pen, taking the inside out to approximate a guide wire and feigning a German accent. "You would think he was delivering a baby." We all die laughing.

Patients for their part were also primed for humor and often made clinical jokes about their own suffering.

> A young woman with KS in her lymph nodes arrives. She and Dr. P jokingly argue. Dr. P looks at her blood work and proclaims in one of his very few Setswana phrases, "Go botoka!" (It is better!). But the patient replies by correcting his pronunciation in a play on words. "No, go botlhoko!" (No, it is painful!). Then she cracks up, and so does Dr. P. She is in pain, but her blood is better—much better. Afterward, Dr. P says to me that she is an example of someone whose expectations are too high.
>
> A middle-aged man (his sister is a nurse at PMH, but she is not with him today) comes into the clinic and sits and shows his arm, which is painful. The chemo infiltrated the vein, which is quite destructive, since it is cytotoxic. It has produced an ugly black mark, but fortunately no open sore. Dr. P jokes with him: "But the tumor is much better, right? You are like someone who comes in with a big huge tumor that we fix and then complain, 'But, doctor,

I now have this little tiny itch on the sole of my foot.'" The patient laughs. "No, the tumor is much better, but the medicine that cured it did this to my arm." Dr. P says, "You know what I like to do to people who complain—to the end of the queue!" The patient laughs and repeats Dr. P's words: "Yes, the tumor is much better."[25]

Yet making cancer biomedically intelligible in this way is tenuous and sometimes disappointing.

Dr. P has a debate with a patient who came yesterday. He says he is not better. Dr. P looks in his mouth, and the tumor is much smaller. But it has left a big hole.

What is efficacy here? Many patients emerged from oncology disfigured and debilitated. For others, focusing on the mass led them to refuse further intervention after the mass had shrunk. Women with breast cancer whose tumors had been downsized might refuse the planned mastectomy. For others, cancer was never adequately enacted, its boundaries never fully sealed. After a miserable cycle or two of chemotherapy, they would return to the *ngaka* (Setswana doctor) or the healing prophet, but not to the ward. "Whatever happened to the woman from Barclays Bank with the KS in her lungs?" we would ask one another. "Can she still be alive?" Often such people would reappear suddenly, some three or six months later, now suffering from a massive recurrence of disease. Having earned the new label of defaulter, they incurred Dr. P's wrath for having vacated the efficacy of his treatment.

On the other hand, there were patients nearing the end of the treatment pipeline who emerged bruised and battered for the journey, but also with some small but growing hope for the fullness of the future. In June 2008 I became a human calendar. I had been away from the ward for a full year. On my first day back in the clinic, Mosadi, whose sister-in-law had seen her deformed breast and brought her in for care—the same Mosadi who had joked about the chemo making her pubic hair fall out—arrived for her clinic appointment. I had been there the year before as she wept on the walk to the surgeons who would amputate her breast and as she vomited into a wad of paper towel after her chemo injections. And now here I was again, many months later, as she returned for a check-up, her radiation, chemo, and surgery completed. She smiled and greeted me, remarking that I had been away for some time. "It's been a whole year," I told her. Then I asked how she was. "A year? A whole year? How am I? I am ALIVE," she said, slowly and deliberately, like it was just dawning on her. "I AM ALIVE." We both sat smiling broadly, enjoying the moment.

Cancer is crystallizing as a fraught bodily and existential experience for individual patients even as it is emerging as an epidemic within Botswana society. This process of emergence merges language, techno-scientific practice, and embodied experience to create the particularities of cancer in Botswana, as distinct from and yet part of the global experience of the disease. Patients are caught between their hopes for efficacy, their need for but wariness of trusting clinical staff, and their increasing physical desperation, a position that efficacious treatment could solve. Yet what is efficacy in this complex world of ideas and differently imagined futures? What is care in this overloaded hospital a decade and a half into a profound AIDS epidemic?

Amputation Day at
Princess Marina Hospital

"It's Amputation Day at PMH!" I wrote in my field notes at some point just after lunch one day in June 2008.[1] By that point, there had been too much amputation talk for one day in this small oncology ward—too many breasts, legs, feet, and testicles to be removed, too much abstraction, cajoling, rot, angst, and loss. The amputation talk had begun first thing in the morning, before ward rounds. I'd been accompanying Dr. P, on his way to check on cancer patients in the medical and surgical wards. We ran into Dr. L. He told Dr. P, "No, I have amputated that KS leg—she bled like a bitch." He looked at me: "Excuse the expression." I do. "But you must do something about this KS," he continued. "I am becoming known as the hindquarter man. And I don't like it."*

Amputation talk had continued through the morning, as we brought women to the surgical clinic to consult about the feasibility of mastectomies. These were quick consultations, with the doctors mainly talking to each other, as the women sat there with breasts exposed. Later, we saw an elderly man whose testicles had been amputated in an effort to halt his prostate cancer. This castration had bought him some extra two years of life, but now we explained to his son that the disease had metastasized to his liver and gut. Amputation talk progressed in the afternoon with failed efforts to convince a man to give up his dead foot. It came to a crescendo with tears, fist pounding, icy silence, and eventually laughter, as a forty-nine-year-old woman struggled to convey the impossibility of being footless. Oncology may lie on the cutting edge of biomedicine, but one of its most fundamental modes of intervention — cutting — is as crude as it comes.

Although I had scrawled "It's Amputation Day at PMH!" in my notebook in black pen, underlining it again and again, in frustration, as the day wore on it wasn't so different from many other days in PMH oncology. Amputation is yet another one of those facets of cancer medicine that is so extraordinary for the patient, yet somewhat routine (if intense) for the clinical staff. Amputation was a clinical problem for Dr. P. Social and psychic complexities might impede his ability to carry out clinical logics, but the imperative of saving or extending life drove his decision-making. Dead feet, dead breasts, rotting penises needed to be removed. Gangrene was a real threat. Metastatic spread needed to be halted. Testes needed to be removed to cut off the hormonal supply that fed prostate cancers.

For patients, amputation was much more than a clinical problem. Rumors circulated among older women in Gaborone that if you went to PMH with cancer, the doctors would amputate your breast and you would die. Often there was truth in the temporal logic of this rumor, of course, but not in its implied causality. Many women came to PMH only when their breasts were so mangled, so painful, that they themselves finally wished it off even if that meant death. For others, losing a leg posed frightening economic, practical, and social prospects. While at PMH, I often wished for a psychologist, a counselor, a therapist, a social worker, someone whose intimacy was professional, someone to protect and heal the psyches of those who had just gone or might soon go under the knife, and perhaps even the saw. But all counseling in this crowded public hospital seemed to take place at the HIV clinics. Global health programs have made what Nancy Hunt and Vinh-Kim Nguyen call "technologies of confession" central to HIV.[2] But these therapeutic modes do not extend into the belly of the hospital.

Relatives often took part in conversations about the need for amputation — but not always. Urging a younger sister to give up a leg, explaining to a father why the doctor wants to castrate him, and supporting a wife whose breast must come off are incredibly difficult forms of intimacy — they reveal the moral stakes of trust. Unlike the doctor, the relative must not only be correct in their recommendation to amputate or not, but he or she had also to live out a commitment to care for the patient in the long-term aftermath of the decision. These are economic, social, emotional, and moral commitments, and they must occur in a complex social world, where lives are deeply intertwined in households and families.

Perhaps the most difficult conversations around amputation involved patients whose legs were plagued with osteosarcoma, a bone cancer that unfortunately most often afflicted teenagers. In PMH, admission to the adult (as versus the pediatric) ward began at age thirteen, so osteosarcoma patients were often the youngest residents of the oncology ward. During the time I spent in the ward, there were numerous cases of fatal osteosarcoma. Because of the relative efficacy of amputation combined with adjuvant chemotherapy, Dr. P, the nurses, Dr. A, and the other medical officers understood these dead or dying teenagers, these marvelous children, to be lost to their families' lack of courage.

In one family, for example, the mother and father initially disagreed over the decision to amputate, and the mother and her relatives, who advocated against amputation, prevailed. This was perhaps because the mother felt more strongly in her convictions against than the father did in favor of the operation. In a world of uncertainty, it is hard to argue forcefully for cutting off your son's leg. What if you are wrong? Indeed, chemotherapy began to shrink the swelling in the boy's femur, and the mother appeared to be vindicated. But within months, just as Dr. P had predicted, the tumor returned ferociously, with metastatic deposits littering the boy's lungs. The uncles came and agreed to the amputation, as the parents sat silently. But Dr. P told them with great bitterness, "No, it is too late now, this disease has spread." The father began to drink heavily. The parents split up. More chemotherapy followed, and the boy, sidelined from the decision but fully aware of its gravity, sat bent over and vomiting from cisplatin—a fifteen-year-old boy in a ward full of men. His mother was now loathed by the staff, and she could barely look her boy in the eye; instead, she spent much of the visiting hour on the female side of the ward, chatting with the relatives of a patient she knew.

Dr. P was haunted. He began to say, "The next time, I am going to court, to get custody. I won't let someone else kill their child in my ward." Dr. A said, "No, I will join you." It was against this background of lost children, and the slipping away of one very beloved boy amid a crumbling family, that the following scene erupted. I had just returned from lunch, and Dr. P brought me into the treatment room to counsel a family, then lost his temper with them. It had been a very stressful day. Dr. P was handling everything alone—the clinic, the ward, the chemo. Dr. A had worked the night shift in anesthesiology directly after his oncology shift the day before, so Dr. P had sent him home that morning after rounds. Dr. E was absent as well, for she was nauseous from taking the prophylactic ARV regimen she required after being stuck by a needle in the chemotherapy room.

In the treatment room, the older sister was doing the talking. The patient, a sixteen-year-old girl with osteogenic sarcoma, sat quietly, with her crutches leaning against the chair in the corner next to the sink. Her mother and aunt were also there. Dr. G, the orthopedic surgeon had sent them to Dr. P because the family wanted to send a report to South Africa for a second opinion before amputation. Dr. P was not a surgeon; when he thought amputation was indicated, he would bring the patient to the surgical clinic for consultation. If the surgeon agreed that the operation was indicated and feasible, the patient would be booked for surgery— and presumably told more about the operation by the surgical staff. But a request for a second opinion was often how a process of hedging on the urgently necessary surgery began. So Dr. G, a kind man who was usually well liked and trusted by his patients (as I knew from my previous research on disability), had no doubt sent the family to Dr. P, hoping that Dr. P could convince them to hurry, and to ultimately opt for the surgery.

Dr. P was enraged and began yelling. He told the family about other families that had pursued second opinions. It was as if he were reliving the death of every child in his head. "You must choose! Leg or life!"* "We do choose life—but amputation is very hard—we care for our small sister, and we want to be sure before we cut."* He railed against them again: "You haven't the right to decide this. This happens every time, and then you will be back in two months begging me to amputate, but it will be too late then."* The sister was also upset. She said, "No, we *do* have the right, the right to be sure and take care of our daughter." At one point, I made eye contact with the patient, and we both smiled. I wondered what she would say if given the opportunity to speak on her own behalf. But this is not the way such decisions are made in Botswana, in PMH, or in a private home. (It also wasn't the way decisions were made in the United States when I was a teenager in the 1980s.) Dr. P said, "And this business where you think that to be disabled is worthless is a disaster."* He was furious. So was the sister.

After he left the room, I confirmed to the sister that she had what she needed to send for a second opinion (pathology report and X-ray), but if she wanted to do it, she must do it immediately. But one of the nurses got upset and picked up where Dr. P had left off. She said, "No! This cancer is too serious, it doesn't wait for weeks or even days—you must do this *ka speed*. If it is invasive, you will have killed your sister." ("wow," I wrote across the top of my notebook, stunned by the nurse's directness.) Then she softened and said, "And you will see this other girl with osteosarcoma walking around the ward on her crutches. Amputation is not so bad, and there are all kind of prostheses." "No," the sister replied, "we are not ashamed to have a sister who is disabled. But we do have to be sure before we do the cutting."

What are patients and staff and relatives to do when they are thrust into relations of intimacy in situations where the stakes are high but the time to develop true trust is lacking? How might an ad hoc trust work, and how might it develop into real trust over time? Amputation is a moment when the tremendously social nature of the human body as experienced outside the clinic comes up against the individuated body that biomedicine takes as its object. It is a moment when decisions hinge on sacrificing a part of the body in the hope of cure, time, or relief. That some of these body parts are dead or dying only adds to the disorienting nature of the experience. The urgency and severity of amputation, the starkness of what it means, lay bare these questions in a painfully direct manner. Amputation shows how such questions are further entangled with those of efficacy, and how impossible it is to extract one life, one body, one person from the others in which it is enmeshed, even as amputation's psychic and bodily horrors reveal the profound boundaries of the human body. In the moment of the cutting, the patient will be quite alone on the table.

Let me offer you one more story as an ethnographic gesture toward the ways that trust and intimacy are shot through with ethical dilemmas, pragmatics, and affect—layers not readily disentangled. It is the final one in my notebook from that entry on "amputation day at PMH."

> In the chemo room, Dr. P has failed to convince a man with a foot that is rotting from KS [to agree] to the amputation. The man is on crutches, the foot is dead, it can no longer bear much weight. But he was appalled at the suggestion he give it up, and the sawing motion Dr. P made did not help to sugarcoat the reality. As the patient sat there waiting for the nurse to clean and bandage it, we crossed the hall to the clinic room to see the final patient of the day.

A woman with a massive sarcoma in her foot arrives with a nurse from Kanye. The thing is absolutely enormous and necrotic. It is incredible. Dr. P takes a photograph. [When I looked at it later, on my hard drive, I noticed she was wearing a green string from a healing church at her ankle.] Then he goes to do a fine-needle aspiration. She is a large woman, arrived with a tukwi [headscarf] wrapped around her foot. She is from a village to the west and is wearing a white sweater and a denim skirt. When Dr. P does the procedure, the thing REALLY *bleeds. Susan runs to get gauze and gloves, with blood pouring onto the floor. I follow up with more. Dr. P asks Dr. M to come and put a cannula in, in case she needs fluid. The bleeding stops. Dr. P says, "OK, you need to get used to the idea that this thing has to come off." He says that this must happen at her leg at the ankle. He makes a sawing motion with his hand. "It must come off or it will kill you." The nurse from her local primary hospital who has accompanied her says, "Well, she knows, but she has been refusing it." It turns out this has been going on for a year or two.*

*The patient says she needs to ask her parents. She is forty-nine years old. Dr. P says, "*NO*, it must come off or you will die." At one point the patient says, "No, you are a very aggressive man. Why is this man so aggressive?"*

Dr. P walks out, and I look at her and say, "Go bokete" [This is heavy], and she begins to cry. I come with tissues and also rub her back. Susan walks in, and it is the three of us in the room huddled together. The patient says, "No, my child cannot walk. My child cannot hear. What can happen if I too am disabled?" Dr. P walks back in, and we explain the situation to him. In fact, we have something of an argument. . . .

Dr. P says it must come off! The woman says, "Ke a utlwa! Ke a utlwa!" [I understand, I feel, I hear—think of the double meaning]. But she must talk to her parents. "No, this is YOUR *decision. Your parents are not doctors. How can they decide? This is for doctors to decide—this is cancer!" I say, "Yes, you must be an expert in cancer—but are you going to be there to take care of her when she comes home from the hospital? When she cannot work!"*

"There are prostheses," Dr. P says. It continues in this way. The patient is now pissed off (as Susan says). But eventually Dr. P says, "OK, then bring your parents to the Kanye hospital and let them talk to the doctors."

*As she is leaving, we have some joking—about what I cannot remember—and she laughs. The nurse is good. This is not a wealthy woman. Afterward, Dr. P comes back in, and we have a vigorous debate. I, too, might have yelled. He says, "*NO*, the bottom line is that I get more patients to*

agree to these amputations on time than someone like Dr. G with his soft approach. You think I am too hard on them, but I have a higher success rate."
"No, no, this woman or that man over there"—I gesture across the hall to where the man with the dead foot, yellow-and-black-spotted like a rotting banana skin, sits—"they are adults. There is a person in that leg! You must have dialogue. It is not hard or soft, but dictatorial or angry, or in dialogue, taking the person seriously." We are left in disagreement. But Dr. P does have a point. It is a burden to be able to see someone's future when they refuse it, even if they refuse it because this future is full of impossibilities. Hard or soft, leg or life is a real choice.

And sometimes in fact, it was Dr. P's impassioned bluntness that inspired trust in the end, once the shock of his manner wore off, once the patient accepted that this aggressiveness meant that he was willing to be the bad guy, to be despised, to be relentless in order to preserve life. It marked his unambiguous morality, his trustworthiness in the face of the most intimate of decisions.

Perhaps you heard echoes of the colonial hospital, with its perverse power relationships.[3] Serious illness is a profoundly vulnerable state, and public institutions are intimidating and disciplining spaces. But Dr. P's aggression is not born of extreme social distance from his patients. Nor is he abusive or sadistic. Batswana relatives and patients alike are self-determined people. They may not yell, but they are not easily pushed around. Perhaps doctors cannot yell like this in an American hospital, but they can be coldly indifferent to the patient, wholly detached.

Amputation, of course, is not a day. It is much longer than that. Some patients and some relatives held fast to their decisions and their body parts. The yelling, the threats of death were for naught, though the deaths themselves were all too real. There were even one or two patients who rebounded despite refusing the amputation, patients to whom Dr. P would say, "Just look at you. You were right, I wanted to take that leg off, but you are getting some motion out of it now!" And amputations, of course, are not without risk. But there were also quite a few patients for whom the memories of blunt talk and even of yelling were now emplotted in broader experiences of healing, however incomplete. Many arrived at a state of great relief to have finally shed a rotting part, even if they had to be pushed there by an aggressive doctor. There were even patients, now disfigured but hale, who joked with Dr. P about the arguments they had

had, who made fun of his dramatic gestures, all of which now were just another facet of their mutual commitment to one another—doctor and patient. Surely there were others for whom the trauma of the argument punctuated the pain of their loss.

Not all days were so stressful or so short-staffed. And there were multiple conversations with relatives and patients about these operations, for these were decisions that were made in stages. Ultimately, no surgery could proceed without the consent of patients (or, in the case of minors, of parents or guardians). But if cancer is about life and death, it is also about gradations of such, about the deaths of parts that sustain life. And in a cancer ward, no less than in a family home, the ghosts of past patients, past decisions, past mistakes sometimes crowd the living as clinicians, nurses, relatives, and even patients try to redeem past losses, past mistakes by rewriting the future.

FOUR

The Moral Intimacies
of Care

Moral sentiment and political efficacy are fragile in ways carefully revealed in the intimacies of care. Care-giving in PMH oncology takes on a particular moral urgency for two reasons. It does so, first, because of the nature of oncology as a body of practice. Oncology is a domain of medicine where harming continually threatens healing in disorienting ways, for oncological therapeutic practices consist of poisoning, burning, and cutting. Care-giving is morally pressing, second, because in a cancer ward, to follow Solzhenitsyn's classic insight, we see clearly how health instantiates politics. Botswana's program of universal care is in keeping with a public political narrative in which Botswana's success is rooted in an enduring history of participatory democracy stretching back to precolonial times, a political philosophy centering around the concept of *botho* (African humanism), and where the circulation of collective wealth mediates hierarchies of class and status.[1] This narrative is overly nostalgic, yet the existential, social, and political import of such health policy is made clear in the shadow of the profound AIDS epidemic that has shaken Botswana to its very foundations over the past decade and a half.[2] The social and political nature and thereby the moral stakes of healing are never more evident than in these periods of intense collective vulnerability, when the weight of survival threatens to overwhelm the processes of care and the webs of relationships that sustain communities.[3]

Policing the critical moral boundary between harming and healing, mediating the relationship that is cancer in this ward, caring for one's fellow human beings (botho) is the work of a small group of nurses and their partners in care — patients.[4] Their political philosophy is embodied, heartfelt, and articulated. Like all philosophies, its ideals are often subverted amid the ebb and flow of daily life. The moral sentiments of the nurses and patients are enacted in terms of professionalism, citizenship, and religiosity.[5] Nurses and patients alike are generally Christian. Though they actively affiliate (or don't) with a variety of churches and denominations, on some level they share a Christian-inflected moral framework of care and spiritual strength. As a philosophy of social healing, nursing is highly contextual.

DEATH OF A MEMBER OF THE WARD

20 May 2009

Mma S arrives for the night shift. It is my first time to see her since returning to PMH oncology this year. We have a nice long chat. Eventually she turns to the bad news she has to tell me. Ticky is late. [Ticky was a wonderful young woman with a rare blood cancer, who had been a regular in the ward for several years.] Now Ticky's father has colon cancer. I had never known, but it turns out that Mma S and Ticky were relatives. Here is what Mma S told me.

"Dr. P was in Germany last year, visiting his mother, and it must have been shortly after he left. Dr. P likes his work too much, and he will even call when he is away in Germany and ask about this patient and that one. So Ticky was here, and she started bleeding. The disease converted and took a bad turn. She was critically ill, she was O positive, and there was no blood at PMH so we called GPH — also no blood, and we were so worried! So Dr. M called Dr. P in Germany, and from there he said, 'No, we MUST get her the blood!' So he called South Africa and arranged for blood that side, and they drove it to the border and he said, 'No, they will call you when it gets there.' And they called and one of the nurses went to the border to get it. Six, we gave her six units of O positive, but still she was bleeding everywhere, and she was asking for Dr. P. And we said, 'No, he is at home,' but then when the plane landed he came straight here. And she was bleeding everywhere and couldn't see because of it, but we said, 'No, he is here,' and she started calling out — from right there" — she points to the female A cubicle of beds. "'Mma J, I am dying! Mma S, I am dying!' Calling to us nurses, and we

came, and she called for Mma T, so we ran to male medical ward [where Mma T had been reassigned] to get her and brought her here. And Dr. P was crying, and she died then with Mma T holding one hand and Dr. P the other. And we, all of us, we were crying. When the shift ended, we did not leave. Dr. M and Dr. S and Dr. P and the nurses; we just sat here crying. These things, this disease it is too cruel. HIV is better than cancer—you can take those ARVs, you will be fine. But cancer, it is too cruel. You tell me, tell me, tell me—when will there be a cure for cancer? When will there be new treatments?" This was one of the most heartfelt pleas for scientific progress I think I've ever heard.

Cancer is a terrible thing. The patients lying in the beds of PMH oncology are very sick. Some have open necrotic wounds. Others have pressure sores. Still others suffer open sores in their mouths or anuses from radiotherapy. Some are hooked up to intravenous drips of cytotoxic chemicals that produce profound nausea and diarrhea. Others can no longer swallow, their throats blocked with esophageal tumors that force them to spit their saliva into a wad of paper towel every few minutes. Many are in tremendous pain. Some are disfigured by disease and surgery. Some have catheters or tracheostomies or colostomies to manage. All are worried, many are bored, some are depressed. Some patients have mothers or sisters or aunts who come to care for them in the evenings, helping to bathe and feed them. Some have family, friends, church members, and colleagues who visit them and call their cell phones. Many others are far from home. Some are dying. All of them need care.

The nurses broker this terrible thing, cancer. Their job is an intensely important one, and an extremely difficult one. They do not always succeed. This chapter examines the stakes and processes of their work, tacking back and forth between ethnography and explication. Nursing is a remarkably complicated endeavor at PMH, one best understood by situating nurses fully in the structural, social, moral, and often pressing existential realities of their working lives.[6] After clarifying the features of nursing care in the ward, I examine the moral significance of the bodily care that nurses provide, then conclude by looking at the relationships between relatives, patients, and nurses and the ways that nurses extend and reshape social healing within the microcosm of the cancer ward.

THE STAKES OF CARE

Care-giving is a moral endeavor.[7] It is at once deeply personal and deeply social, and it is a vital practical matter, crucial to patient well-being and survival. In the PMH oncology ward, professional care-giving is also an inherently political act. The bodily care Batswana nurses provide is part of a system of universal care in a country that is still in the throes of a widespread and overwhelming epidemic of HIV/AIDS, while also grappling with a rapidly escalating cancer epidemic. Nursing in PMH oncology is an extension of the state's commitment to care for its people, a manifestation of an explicit national ethos of collective care and compassion, and as such it exposes ongoing tensions between personal and state responsibilities and entitlements. Unlike doctoring, which is often performed by expatriates, professional nursing is a Tswana endeavor; and unlike doctoring, which is shielded behind the opacity of scientific expertise, technology, and jargon, nursing work is far more accessible to evaluation by the public.

The past decade and a half has been fraught for the nursing profession in Botswana. Once a prestigious job that presented one of the very few opportunities for upward mobility available to Batswana women, over the past fifteen years nursing has fallen from grace and into a period of ambiguity, even as a shortage of trained nurses has emerged as a major national crisis.[8] In these dynamics, Botswana is far from alone. The "nursing crisis" is a pressing global phenomenon. Yet the shortage of nurses in wealthier countries in turn draws experienced nurses from poorer countries, part of the infamous African "brain drain."[9]

Concern over the quality of nursing and in particular the attitude of nurses in the country is long-standing. But by the late 1990s, as the AIDS epidemic exploded into Botswana's clinics and hospitals, these concerns took on a powerful import. Nurses were regularly characterized in newspapers, in political discussions, and among the general public as callous, rude, uncaring bureaucrats. Such criticisms were matched by equally strong recognition of their importance to the core medical and public-health enterprise of the country.[10] Over the past decade, nurses have organized for better pay, they have gone on strike, they have left for greener pastures, and sadly, they, too, have become patients and died. Perhaps nowhere is this more evident than at PMH. In 2001, at the very pinnacle of the AIDS epidemic, before ARVs arrived, in the months just before the oncology ward opened, the shortage of nurses was so acute that the hospital superintendent was forced to temporarily close two wards of PMH — this in an institution that could hardly afford to *reduce* capacity.[11] By 2004, with all wards again open, the situation nevertheless had yet to substantially improve. Though the hospital's nurse-to-patient ratio was one of the highest in southern Africa, PMH was operating with only a third of its standard nursing staff. The WHO standard of care is one nurse to a maximum of six patients, but as the *Botswana Daily News* reported at the time, "Nurses at Marina say their average is 10, and can go up to 20 in times of crisis. 'We are extremely overworked, but underpaid. It is not easy to attend to patients on the beds, on the floors, on the trolleys and in cubicles. The wards are always flooded with people, yet there are so few of us,' said a nursing sister."[12] Yet it is also the centrality of their work and the seeming clarity of their mission that opens nurses to such strident criticism.

So, too, nurses have long enjoyed the privileges of gate-keeping, wielding as they do tremendous, if quotidian, power over the fortunes of those who seek their care and attention, and over allied workers, including doctors who rely on their labor. In short, nursing is a dangerous endeavor for all involved, highlighting as it does the vulnerabilities of the ill and the frail, and the pettiness on which all bureaucracies feed. Yet, like many such high-stakes endeavors, the potential payoffs are tremendous. When done well, nursing — with its touching, feeding, bathing, listening, noticing — concretizes the humanistic promise of medicine. When shirked or performed as just another bureaucratic function, it concretizes the immorality, the coldness of modern institutions.

Perhaps more than doctoring, nursing is understood to require sentimental work. Compassion, care, empathy, even love are expected to animate and orient the work of nursing, and this is where it seems the greatest critiques lie.[13] Patients, family members, doctors, and the general public alike do not always see the sentimental work they expect from the nurses in PMH. Oncology is unique in the hospital for the rigor with which Dr. P manages bed-space in the ward, but also for the ways the disease and its cyclical management produce long-term relationships between patients and the cancer nurses.

Throughout my research, I met many patients who praised the oncology nurses for their care and support — patients like Ticky, who called for the nurses by name in moments of terrible fear and anguish. I also met patients and relatives who complained bitterly about their needs being ignored or rebuffed by the nurses. It seemed that for every patient or relative who complained about care on the ward, there were many others who praised the nurses, who carried the matron's cell phone number in their pocket and rang her—even in the middle of the night—if there were problems.

Such are the contradictions of oncology nursing in PMH. My point here is neither to valorize nurses nor to condemn them. Many of them are doing extraordinary work under remarkably difficult conditions. It was Mma C from oncology and her nursing colleagues in the surgical wards who of their own initiative, pushing against a thick bureaucracy, began an ostomy clinic to support patients whom they saw emerging from surgery disfigured and lacking support for the management of their new bodily state. On the other hand, some nurses are domineering or lazy, like Mma P, who in 2007 ran the bookings in gynecology in an abusive and rude manner, intimidating patients and staff alike.[14] Sometimes a nurse in oncology would stay long after his shift had ended, simply to see a patient through a bureaucratic challenge, or to assist in a difficult procedure. Other times a nurse might be busy playing solitaire on the ward computer and fail to see a patient in need of assistance at the far end of the ward. Sometimes a nurse would advocate for a patient's humanity, as when Mma C scolded Dr. P for exposing Ninki's cancerous vulva to twelve pairs of eyes during a training round. Other times a nurse would oppose Dr. P in an effort to police her own professional autonomy, even when this went against a patient's interests. I dare say a similar range might be found in *any* workplace—including my own. Yet the stakes here are extremely high, and the work extremely difficult, given the charge of nurses to care for very sick and therefore very vulnerable people in an overcrowded and in some ways dysfunctional institution.[15]

For patients and nurses alike, the cancer ward is both a self-contained institutional space, and one that is porous and connected to home in troubling ways. One of the nurses I worked with in 2006, Mma Z, often seemed detached and was desperate to get transferred to a new ward when the rotations came the following May. It turned out that this was because her mother had previously died in the ward, and it was very difficult for her to spend each day in this place that she hated for its terrible memories of suffering and loss. One cold July day, I watched as another nurse, Rra D, had to leave the clinic and stand outside for a moment to collect himself after a difficult prognostic conversation with a patient, Jane, and her partner, Roger. Both were close childhood friends of Rra D, and Jane, though not yet thirty years old, had just been diagnosed with an extremely aggressive breast cancer. Botswana is a small country, and such moments where home floods into work are not uncommon.

Many nurses, of course, are patients themselves. Some have HIV, others have breast cancer, or diabetes, or hypertension, their privacy potentially compromised by their work. Some nurses (particularly women) were not only taking care of dying or profoundly ill patients in the ward, but also of dying or profoundly ill relatives in their homes each day after their shift in PMH ended. They were expected by their families to be the advocates and brokers for sick relatives who arrived in Gaborone needing care. For families struggling to provide care for the sick, nurses in the family are often the obvious choices, because of their knowledge and skills, because of their assumed resources (after all they are employed), and—when hospitalization or outpatient consultation was a possibility—because of their residential proximity to PMH. Furthermore, their bureaucratic knowledge of the system and their sociological knowledge of the various hospital personnel were recognized as invaluable to patients facing admission to a very challenging institution. But brokering between family and work is far from easy. One nurse from the men's orthopedic ward—a senior and very important nurse—faced the shame of coming to oncology with her brother, a cancer patient, who wore the orange pajamas and shackles that clearly identified him as a prisoner. She looked immensely grateful when Dr. P took the opportunity to lecture her brother sternly on how difficult this was for his sister.

Other times, nurses decide not to reveal these connections publicly because they fear this might complicate matters, making others feel they are playing favorites. Mma S, for example, was related to her patient, Ticky, though I did not learn this until after Ticky's death. Mma S was not alone. It was not until Boitumelo died on the ward that I learned she was the matron's cousin. The following year that same matron lost her brother and returned to the ward after his funeral, only to leave the next day in tears and shock over the unexpected death of her beloved niece. In other words, in addition to the pressures and responsibilities of balancing family and work, some of the nurses in PMH oncology are themselves grieving—and they are grieving in a world where that fact has lost some of its cachet given the overwhelming burden of grief in the country.

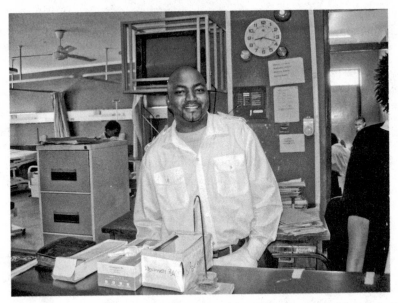

Rra D at the nurses' station. Look at the clock and the spike on the desk. It is just past 8 AM, and already twenty-one patients are in the queue.

Given the nature of their jobs, nurses grieve, of course, not only for lost kin. Many nurses develop deep feelings for some of their patients, whom they come to befriend over the months and years of their illnesses. As Mma D said to me one afternoon, exhausted and reflective at the end of a long day,

> Eh! This disease—this cancer is so terrible. The things it does to people. This place is awful. I don't like working in this ward. You meet patients. You get to know them. You become friends, and then you watch them deteriorate and die. When they die it is your friend. It is too, too, too painful! You see people. They come to the clinic and you see them come there and then eventually you see them start to waste away and enter the agony of it. No, it is just too painful. I hate it here. We grow to love our patients only to watch them die. They become like our family. There are days when it is just so painful for us.*

Of course, not every nurse is like Mma D, willing to undergo this pattern of love and loss over and over and over again. There are certainly some nurses in PMH oncology who appear at times to be disconnected from human suffering. I doubt they were always this way. More likely, the job, the epidemic, the bureaucracy finally eroded their emotional commitment, rendered it unsustainable, perhaps replacing it with depression or anger or indifference.[16] Nonetheless, this presents terrible problems for the patients in their care. And not every patient is like Ticky. Most of the patients in the ward are gracious, polite, humorous, and kind with the nurses and with one another. But occasionally the ward houses a loathsome character, demanding, self-important, obstinate, or lecherous. Yet that person, too, needs and deserves care.

ONCOLOGY AS A SLICE OF THE NATIONAL CAKE

In the PMH oncology ward the promise of citizenship is manifest in access to novel technologies increasingly understood as necessary to collective health and well-being. Nursing is the moral face of citizenship in Botswana's system of universal care—one of the critical ways that patients and relatives understand and evaluate the political promise of care, and the ethics of distribution in a new regime of highly technologized medicine.[17]

The vast majority of PMH nurses and patients are Batswana. By contrast, though there is a small but growing group of Batswana clinicians, particularly medical officers (like Dr. R), most of the doctors in PMH are expatriates. That nurses are almost exclusively Batswana complicates their relationship to PMH in multiple ways, since they are at once employees, past and future patients, advocates for relatives, cultural brokers, and guardians of a very precious form of medical citizenship, even as they occupy a relatively weak position within the institutional hierarchy. It means that many nurses accept their work as civil servants as necessarily about controlling access to resources, often envisioned as a "national cake" that must be shared out equally. And it means that nurses must do a tremendous amount of linguistic and cultural brokering between expatriate doctors and patients.

Botswana is both remarkably hierarchical and also remarkably egalitarian, and this political, social, and cultural formulation combines with a political and economic structure and discourse that treats the bulk of the nation's vast diamond wealth as collective property. Batswana envision national resources as much more of an immediate zero-sum enterprise than Americans like myself do. In the United States we continually defer debt to future generations, sustained by a progressive vision of increasing wealth. Even now, when the current economic situation is dire, for many it is assumed to be temporary if painful.

The Botswana government does not incur debt in this way, and so they have spared their citizens the predations of structural adjustment. In Botswana—bordered as it is by Zambia and Zimbabwe, both of whose amazingly fertile and promising development trajectories were subject to sudden and seemingly long-term if not permanent reversals, on a continent where Botswana is very much the exception that proves the rule— no one assumes that wealth will continue to grow.[18] Borrowing against the national future is recognized to be a foolish game.[19]

While Batswana understand, appreciate, reinforce, and live with all sorts of hierarchies, where the national cake is concerned it is considered extremely problematic if someone receives more than her share. Batswana have long-standing forms of allocation, from the doling out of food at weddings to the sharing out of gifts by returned migrant workers, that are intended to mediate potential tensions between equity and equality.[20] In situations in Botswana where equity is meant to hold, it is less that individuals are expected to mediate their own desires to take too much; instead, institutional practices are recognized as necessary to ensure equity. When I bring chocolates to the ward as a gift, two nurses take them, count them carefully, divide them by the number of staff, then present each staff member with their share. They do not put them out in a bowl and let people help themselves, as might happen back in New York, where I bought them.

Such habits are the result not only of less relative wealth than in the United States, but also of a collective ethos that provides for the kind of healthcare rationing and equitable distribution that Americans have been unwilling to commit to (which has caused tens of millions of U.S. citizens to be consigned to serious healthcare anxieties, deficiencies, dangers, and crushing health-related personal debt). Batswana will not allow this. These habits, too, are the product of a context where corruption is the most feared specter, given the notoriety of corruption on the African continent. These sensitivities to equity and corruption combine with the kind of institutional record-keeping that hospitals excel at in their accounting for resources. Within PMH, the bureaucracy of the state combines with the bureaucracy of the hospital, which combines with cultural forms of equity in distribution. All these operate in a place that is intimate enough to make collectivity palpable, and where nurses as citizens are highly invested in that collectivity. Nurses therefore do see themselves as particularly suited—indeed, they are charged—to carefully watch the dispensing of resources in an institution where the pharmacy, the prescription pad, and the admission form (in short, the national cake) are all by and large controlled by expatriates. This is bound to produce problems.[21]

Nurses in oncology who take pity on, say, an elderly woman after a push injection of doxorubicin and cisplatin must either furtively offer her a red biohazard bag to help her contain her vomit while she travels to the bus rank for her journey home, or develop steely countenances and pretend not to see her predicament. This is a difficult decision, especially after it has been stressed in circulars and meetings that the biohazard bags are scarce and not to be given out.[22] It also means that sometimes a nurse will wield a petty form of power by fetishizing bureaucratic details—access to supplies, appointments, bed-space, and patient queues—in ways that make little sense in terms of care, but which condense moral judgments over the deserving or undeserving nature of particular patients or their familial caregivers. Such judgments were sometimes wielded against relatively wealthy patients and their relatives, who were often more agentive about their needs and vocal in their opinions about care, and whom nurses might perceive as taking resources they could and should provide themselves. It also means that many nurses are hemmed in both by a form of medical citizenship and by the realities of expatriate doctoring, such that they themselves (their labor and their moral sentiment) are a part of the national cake to be allocated. In other words, patients and their relatives might complain that they are not getting enough nursing from the state.

These issues are playing themselves out against a shifting epidemiological landscape in PMH that has required nurses to manage crowds on the one hand and to care for very sick people with inadequate resources on the other. The situation is in some way comparable to that of the American teacher in an overcrowded public school who finds herself forced to essentially shift her energies from teaching to policing in her classroom. But in the cancer ward, where bed-space is more tightly managed than in other wards of the hospital, and where many patients become known to staff over the course of their illnesses, moral sentiment and care, while still hard work, are somewhat more easily achieved.[23]

BODY, INTIMACY, HUMAN

At 7:20 AM on an ordinary February day in 2007, the nurses begin their "handover" meeting. Arriving in their pressed white uniforms, with epaulets and pins marking their rank and training, the nurses crowd into the small anteroom at the back of the ward, with its microwave oven, electric kettle, two wooden chairs, and the calendar and "duty rosta" pinned on the wall alongside photographs, postcards, and announcements. Greetings are exchanged, jokes cracked, new hairdos admired. Mma R has a new wig. Mma L has a headache. Mma C makes fun of the rumpled clothing of the visiting ethnographer, whose sorry ironing skills are a source of regular amusement.

When everyone is in the office, seated on counter or chairs, or leaning against the wall, each patient's file is read out, including the doctor's notes and the nursing notes from the previous night and this morning, both handwritten on white paper that has been hole-punched and tied into the file with yarn. Unlike the doctors, the nurses make a serious effort to know all their patients' names, always. Attention is paid to the intravenous lines—how and what to run or finish, which medications have been stopped, which medications have been ordered, problems with pain, constipation, and nausea. Vital signs are read for each patient. Mma T, a senior nurse in her late fifties, her gray hair in small braids, who is just finishing the shift she began alone at 11 the previous night, points out one patient who has been restless with pain, though on codeine phosphate. During the night the medication tended to wear off very quickly, so he will need his pain medicine upped, she explains.

It is very quiet and peaceful on the ward. The patients are sleeping; morning visitors have left. Mma C, the shift manager, assigns the morning nurses to their duties as the ward begins to come to life: Rra D to the clinic, Mma N to accompany patients to radiotherapy at the private hospital across town. Mma N groans; there are four stretcher cases for her to lift. Mma R is asked which beds she wants. She points to the three empty beds in Male A cubicle: "I will take those." Everyone laughs, then Mma C divides the beds up among the three nurses covering the floor. The nurses fan out to greet each of their patients for the morning and begin taking vitals on patients who are now getting their *motogo* (soft sorghum porridge), milk, and sugar from Tiny, the cleaner, who is rolling a metal cart through the ward serving breakfast. The nurses chat and joke with the patients they know.[24]

At approximately 8 AM, the handover completed and Mma T having departed for the bus rank, the nurses come to stand behind the desk in the center of the ward, facing the waiting benches in the corridor, which are now filling up with patients. They are joined by the nursing assistants, who run errands, process clinic paperwork, and do data entry and translation in the clinic. Someone, in an act of Christian charity, grabs the rumpled, tone-deaf ethnographer from where she is sitting and scribbling into her black notebook. Then, lining up in a row, the nurses sing to Jesus. The complex harmonies of Tswana choral music are incredibly rich and beautiful, and they echo down the corridor. The ethnographer lip-synchs with great enthusiasm. Mma S comes out from behind the nurse's station, Setswana Bible in hand, and begins to preach. Her voice feverishly rising and falling, she implores Jesu to heal the sick, to help the patients, to bless the doctors in their work.

Mpho is now sitting up in her bed with her Bible, as is Christine, a forty-year-old woman with breast cancer in the next bed. Patients and relatives sitting on the waiting benches are listening. Mma S offers up the Bible, and Mariana, another patient, takes it and reads a verse. Then there is a final hymn with Mma L, a young nurse with a truly gorgeous voice, who sings out the cues for the next verse. Prayers over, Dr. P and Dr. A arrive and greet the nurses with handshakes, and the ward round is under way.

So begins each day in this cancer ward, as the nurses prepare for clinical work and mark their corner of PMH as a moral space, a place of hope, and courage, and faith. It is hard to stress how important this moment is, each morning, to clarify the purpose of medicine, to remind very sick patients that God is there and that their nurses pray for them. Through their joking, and laughter, and gossip, and occasional strife, nurses also create the ward as an intensely social world. This is a world where apathy and depersonalization continually threaten the moral project—more so, even, than jealousy and competition threaten the morality of the world beyond the hospital walls—yet also where the potential to rehumanize decomposing bodies animates the work at hand.

Professional medical work, as many observers have suggested, is primarily task-oriented. For many nurses in PMH, AIDS has reprioritized tasks, given the high volume of patients, many of whom are very sick. Changing diapers, for example, and, in the oncology ward, emptying the vomitus are perpetual, tedious, and unpleasant tasks. On the occasions when this work is shirked, it is horrible for the patients. Yet nurses are not maids, or cleaners, or porters. For nurses to embrace them professionally, tasks need to be embedded in the care the nurses provide.

Take, for example, a curious debate that emerged one Friday afternoon in oncology in April 2007. It was not unique. I was to witness this same dynamic on more than one occasion. On this day the oncology ward was already overcrowded, with extra beds packed into the female side. Therefore, Naledi, an immobilized breast cancer patient with bone metastases and a passive fracture who needed palliative radiotherapy, had been admitted to the female orthopedic ward while awaiting transfer to oncology. Naledi needed to go to GPH for radiation, and on that day there were already two stretcher cases in female oncology headed to GPH, both of whom were large, heavy women. The orthopedic nurses wanted the oncology nurses to collect Naledi and bring her to GPH with the other two patients. The oncology nurses protested this, arguing that she was not their patient and asking the orthopedic nurses to transport her instead. The orthopedic nurses replied by asking oncology nurses to come to their ward and administer the drugs for this patient.

A huge struggle ensued, at which point Dr. P got involved and made things worse by asking that the orthopedic nurses bring the patient as far as oncology, from where the oncology nurses could bring her to GPH. This solution angered everyone. Finally, an exasperated Dr. P decided, pounding his fist, that, space be damned, Naledi would be transferred to oncology. "Transfer Naledi—we will squeeze her in somehow!" Then he turned to the nurses and pointed out that they had only added to their own workload by refusing to transport her, for now they would need to bathe, medicate, and otherwise care for her as well. Eventually, Naledi was brought to oncology, but too late in the day to make it to radiotherapy. She would have to begin the following week.

Afterward the nurses were very angry about what had happened but, surprisingly enough, were happy about the transfer, even though it meant more work for them. As Mma D said, trying to explain the situation to me, "No, we are not donkeys! Bring the patient here and it will be much better! Let her stay here if she is our patient, and we won't mind." In other words, some tasks (like lifting stretcher cases for transport, or changing

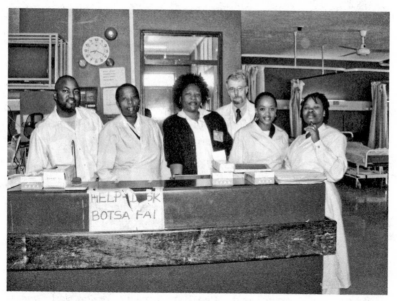

Dr. P and the nurses at the nurses' station.

diapers) may be low status and unpleasant, but once those tasks — or any tasks, even the giving of medicine — are separated from the moral responsibility of care for an individual patient, an "identified life," they also become merely that: tasks, porterage, cleaning, the work of donkeys.[25] But when they are embedded in the flow of care for a human being, those tasks are subsumed within a professional commitment and moral ethos of care and humanization. Unfortunately, Naledi had to wait yet longer for her radiotherapy in order for this point to be made.

If the work of nursing in an overcrowded institution amid simultaneous epidemics of AIDS and cancer threatens to reduce nurses to donkeys, the threat these diseases pose to the humanity of patients is even more acute. The grim fact is that some of Botswana's advanced cancer patients are physically rotting. Their tumors have burst the skin, harnessing and rerouting blood supply for growth in networks that produce tissue death and the deep stink of necrotic flesh. Cleaning such wounds at home, especially in compounds without running water and with only a limited supply of linens and soap, is extremely difficult. And relatives often find it hard to approach such wounds without experiencing palpable fear and disgust, which is understandably troubling to patient and relative alike.[26] It is this rot, and its accompanying stink and sight that in earlier decades made cancer an obscenity in North America and Western Europe. One of the most crucial tasks of oncology nursing is to humanize patients whose bodies are undergoing profoundly disfiguring processes of decomposition. Wound and bodily care for the rotting is a site where the combination of technical skill, professional knowledge, and the sentimental work of cancer nursing concretizes the humanistic promise of medicine.

9 March 2007

Dumisane, the guy with the hole in his head, is here.[27] His blood is OK, so he will have chemo, but first the wound [from the tumor on his neck] has to be cleaned. The nurse who brought him says [in the clinic] at Letlhakeng there were maggots in the wound, and they cleaned it with hydrogen peroxide. It must not have been today, because the bandage is dirty. The nurse is from the health post, and he hasn't seen the wound himself. He runs off when Mma T and I go to clean it. Mma T rolls her eyes. We don plastic aprons, masks, and gloves, and get two dressing packs. The trolley is already in use with another patient. We push Dumisane's gurney into the ward, into Male A cubicle, squeezing it next to bed 5, which we push to the side. We can't use the chemo room, because we will need suction for the maggots. Hydrogen peroxide is not good because it just boils the maggots and leaves them in the wound—dead and rotting—better to vacuum them out and then dress it.

We pull the curtain (but still the man in bed 3 can see in, since the curtain doesn't close all the way). Then I hold the bib—wait, actually first we cut the suction tube with a sterile blade and hold it with sterile gauze waiting and pull the patient up to sitting. Peeling off his long navy raincoat and layers, [we see that] Dumisane is like a skeleton. I am shocked to learn he is only fifty-four years old—he looks like he is in his seventies. I hold the bib and the suction while Mma T removes the gauze. She soaks a lot of cotton in saline and then uses [it] to peel the bandages off because they are all stuck to the wound, so the moisture helps to remove them. She reassures Dumisane, "Sorry, Rra Dumisane, sorry. Sorry, Rra, botlhoko [pain]! Sorry." But he is a quiet man and does not like to talk so much during the cleaning, unlike some patients with whom the exchange is continuous. The wound is ENORMOUS—*open, gaping, and vascular. But there are no maggots. This is good. We can drop the suction and both be on the same side of the patient, with an easier set up. Mma T puts on the sterile gloves and begins to clean with saline, scooping out clots of blood and necrotic tissue, then throwing* the gauze in the biohazard bag as she goes. She doesn't like forceps, they are awkward, she explains—but when a wound is so deep, you need to use them to get all the way in. After the deepest part, she uses her hands for control. She keeps one sterile and one dirty and passes the gauze between—never letting them touch.

I ask her about cleaning someone else's wound. How do you know how gentle or hard you can be? She says, "You learn how to do it, as a student your hand shakes—but as you learn, it stops shaking, and you can do it with confidence, making sure it moves." Dumisane remains completely still, only a few times making an eesh [ouch]. I am holding his shoulders to keep the back of the bib [fashioned from a sterile pad] closed and then cupping the front to catch the blood. He looks sad. I think it is a lonely situation for him, powerless with this stinking horrible thing. When the wound is cleaned, a lot of blood has pooled out onto the bib. Mma T takes it away and begins to pack the wound with gauze that she has soaked in betadine. I hold the soaked pieces of the gauze in place as she adds more layers. The wound is so wide and deep it takes a lot to pack it. Then as I continue to hold the betadine-soaked pack in place, she starts adding dry, clean gauze over it. I try to hold gingerly, but firmly. As the dry, clean gauze is added, it somehow feels good to see it looking so clean and fresh. Mma T asks if it is completely covered—if there is some opening, then it is a pathway for new bacteria to enter. "It needs one more bit of gauze, here." "I'm coming over with it!" And then it is all covered. It takes both of my hands spread wide over his throat to hold it all in place. Then Mma T wraps it with a bandage and puts on the clips. Dumisane asks if he can lay down now, he is so tired, and we say yes. So he is resting with his olive green hat back on his head covering the hole, and navy trench coat. He still has chemo left to go. One of the nurses sprays a blast of cinnamon air freshener.

Mma T reports to Dr. P that there are no maggots—but that soon the wound will be like Kgosietsile's. Kgosietsile's was so big you could see the organs in the neck. This one you can't see yet, but soon you will. She has to remind Dr. P who Kgosietsile was [nurses in oncology always seem to remember patients by their names, while Dr. P remembers each patient by face and condition], then he recalls him. Dr. P says, "I felt so bad then, because even me, I felt such an aversion to that wound. I didn't want to look at it and that was so awful."

Mma T says, "Yes, there were maggots, he could feel them crawling around in there and call us. I was afraid to clean him the first time, but of *course I couldn't dodge. I just said, 'OK, before you assign me to that I want to come and take a look, to know what to expect under that bandage.' So I looked while someone else was cleaning, and I said, 'OK, now I've seen it.' No surprises and the next day, when it was my turn, Mma D assisted me, and it was fine. Then I could do it easily, and Kgosietsile was very lively — even when you were cleaning the wound."*

The care and attention with which oncology nurses clean necrotic wounds and thereby rehumanize patients who have disfiguring growths is extraordinary. Each day outpatients arrive in clinic wrapped in dirty, stinking, often homemade bandages. They leave freshly covered with clean, white cloth. It is a crucial moment of respite on the arduous journey to death. One elderly woman whose entire leg was rotting with malignant melanoma arrived with her daughter, painfully trundling in, with two mop handles as canes, her foot wrapped in a disposable diaper to catch the blood and tissue. When I told Mma F, a very intimidating senior nurse (who later that year would be diagnosed with breast cancer), how impressed I was with the care she brought to the cleaning of this patient's leg — such that the patient and her daughter were both able to laugh and joke during the cleaning — her voice actually cracked and tears came to her eyes. She felt this among the most important work she did in PMH oncology and was touched that someone had noticed. I asked Mma E, another senior nurse, about this as well. She said,

Yes, that is why nurses of all people must have empathy. Not sympathy, not pity, but empathy. You have to really *feel* [*go utlwa*, or to feel, to understand, to sense, to hear] that you want that patient to get better, to feel OK. With experience, you don't feel that sickness or disgust or fear from the wounds. You can't, if you are a nurse. You cannot let the patient feel that you are afraid of them or that you are disgusted by them. If nurses do not do this job, then who will? Who will? The relatives they will feel that fear, OK they may not want to look. It is OK. But we must. When I was training as a nurse, I lost a colleague in the first year that way. We went to learn to dress wounds and that woman couldn't handle it — she dropped out of the program. In my second year the teacher really made sure we saw a patient with rotting cancer of the breast. Two students vomited, and the teacher made them stay for three hours with that vomit. At the time, we all thought that she was being cruel, but now we know she was teaching us something important.

By contrast, on 22 May 2009, a young woman lay dying in the ward with a particularly egregious wound on her neck. Maggots had developed in her wound the previous day, and as I wrote in my notes:

> The new, young, male nurse, Rra K, upon being assigned to her bed says in Setswana, "No, I haven't done this before." And the shift manager, Mma J, says, "You need the heart of a man to do this. It is natural, the fear." And so we all discuss. I say, "You will get used to it, look for a while, to make it familiar." And Rra D says, "No, some things you never get used to." Dr. R agrees.

In other words, cancer nursing is an embodied practice. But it is a fine-tuned form of embodiment. Effective nurses may not be disgusted or afraid such that it might compromise patient care, or such that the patient feels repulsive or shunned or separated from the flow of social experience. Yet there is a danger if one gets so used to the wounds and the agony that one experiences no aesthetic reaction at all. Nurses and clinicians, my friends were saying, should be physically and emotionally moved by the obscenity of cancer, moved to compassionate and practical action. This, too, was a form of empathy.

In practicing empathy within biomedical care, oncology nurses draw on the resources of a collective moral imagination they share with patients, one shaped in part by Setswana and local Christian understanding. Empathy is predicated on a kind of intersubjectivity that is often effaced by or pushed to the background of biomedical ideas and practice, but which is foundational to *bongaka* (therapeutics). Much of bongaka assumes a social permeability of the body, such that the feelings, thoughts, and actions of one person can produce bodily effects in another.[28] Similarly, in their remarkable accounts of various apostolic churches in Botswana, the anthropologists Fred Klaits and Richard Werbner have demonstrated the centrality of empathy to prophetic practices of healing and care for church members.[29] Klaits shows how members of one church continually orient their Christian practice around human reciprocity, which finds expression in part through the moral sentiment in nursing care. Werbner, in a different church, explains how healing hinges on the ability of church prophets to vicariously endure their patients' suffering and thus materialize the patient's interiority in and on their own bodies. The moral philosophy of Batswana nurses, with its emphasis on empathy — on the ability to perceive another's suffering at the level of feeling, and to then in turn transform that suffering by recalibrating their own bodily consciousness — offers deep insights into the intersubjective phenomenology of care.

If such wounds are occasions for the enactment of professionalism and positive moral sentiment in the oncology ward, it is in part because they are an upsetting challenge to the material and moral limits of home-based nursing care. One young woman accompanied her grandmother each week to oncology for blood work and chemotherapy. On several occasions the nurses tried to instruct her on how to clean the wound on her grandmother's cancerous breast. This included using a syringe to get the saline into a deep pocket of infection in the wound, which was appallingly large. The granddaughter was greatly affected by the wound, and her eyes would widen and then avert as she backed out of the clinic office. She found herself unable to help her grandmother tend to this wound, a fact which made her extremely uncomfortable. "Ke a tshaba" (I am too afraid), she whispered to me. "Go ferosa sebete?" (Does it nauseate you?), I whispered back. Yes, she affirmed, nodding her head. She was not alone in this reaction; other relatives struggled with these feelings, too, though many caregivers were able to overcome such aversions.[30]

For the patient, living with this rot and disfigurement is deeply exhausting, among other significant challenges. Flies circle such patients constantly, and the stink can cause others to distance themselves. Not only do nurses reaffirm the humanity of patients who are decomposing, by addressing their wounds matter of factly and gently, but they also constitute the ward as a site of at least partial respite for patients from the energy required to mediate the effects their bodies may have on others. Lying in PMH oncology, finally, at last, one need not worry so much about one's smell, as nurses move about the ward cleaning wounds and blasting air freshener. Patients, too, aided in one another's respite. Indeed, on the occasions when patients had to explain to clinical staff that their nausea was being triggered by smells, they always took care to clarify, loudly, that they were referring to food or chemical smells, ensuring their fellow patients would not feel responsible for the odor of their vomit or rot or diarrhea.

THE AD HOC THERAPY MANAGEMENT GROUP

The PMH cancer ward is an open ward. It is a neighborhood within the strange village that is PMH, and this fact extends the social work of nursing, with its greetings, jokes, prayers, conversation, quarrels, and laughter, as well as the humanizing body work that lies at the core of care. Through the distorting prism of the ward, the therapy management group that John Janzen first described as a cornerstone of African social healing is temporarily reconfigured.[31]

In May 2009 I watched an elderly man rise in his striped pajamas and cross the cubicle to instruct a younger man on how to clean his tracheal tube, just as during clinical rounds I had seen many patients advocate for or explain the circumstances of their neighbors in an effort to improve those people's care. In June 2008 Dr. P temporarily commandeered a cubicle in the eye ward, for five patients (four with cervical cancer, one with breast cancer) who had arrived together from the northern referral hospital for radiotherapy at GPH. Four of these women expressed deep concern over the pain and depression of their neighbor, reporting her distress to the oncology team on rounds and seeking to reassure her as she grappled with the loneliness and fear of being so far from her children for weeks on end. Hospitalization, like serious illness more generally, is a process of social estrangement.[32] But a temporary, condensed, social world is created within the hospital, one with its own personalities, rhythms, attachments, and politics. For some patients, this new neighborhood extends the logics of social healing into the heart of the biomedical institution, mitigating the isolation of illness.

12 March 2007

At lunchtime I go to talk to the man with cancer of the hypopharynx in Male B bed 4. Dr. P asked me to talk to him because he is upset and depressed. How have I become a counselor for the dying? I ask Mma D to come with me, and she does. This man has been told the other day that it is cancer—so he only wants to know if it can be healed. He is depressed. Mma D and I back him up and explain what cancer is—and also how the chemo works. It is cyclical. "You are not being sent away. You will come back in three weeks for more medicine, and then bo-three weeks, three weeks, three weeks, until you have taken the chemo six times." It seems he was worried that he was being sent [home] to Palapye and there would be no more treatment. "Is there anyone at home when you get there?" He is in his fifties—the wife is late, but his mother and kids are there. One is a soldier. He [the patient] describes how it feels when he tries to talk—the tumor grabs him inside the throat. He is worried about his voice. I use the metaphor "bomb" for chemo. I reassure him that the treatment is powerful and the body needs to rest afterward, but that he will come back for the next course of treatment. Mma D and I are trying to make him myopic, to limit his temporal horizon of concern. And I explain [as Dr. P explained to me] how the tumor could shrink quite a bit before he experiences a change in sensation, given where it sits. His prognosis is terrible, and we don't tell him this. I think he knows. Words can kill. But we encourage him to focus on each day rather than worrying about a future that only God knows, and to have patience.

We three grope for a pathway out of his existential angst. Then we find it—over there in the opposite bed! He begins gossiping with us about the man with cancer of the esophagus from Mahalapye—the one whose wife is always here helping him. He says, with a knowing smile, "That man always wants the wife around, near him. Because he is older than her and afraid she will sleep with another man." Then he starts laughing with us about it, going into more detail and is greatly cheered up—but I am so worried that we gave him false hope.

As in all neighborhoods in Botswana, relatives come to visit. They cycle in and out of the ward during prescribed visiting hours, though some patients come from far, and thus not every bed is surrounded by family. Several years ago a friend told me the following story. Her brother-in-law, Wabona, had been in PMH oncology with cancer. He was required to provide a consent form, for a surgical procedure, that his wife, Tshepiso, had to sign. Although PMH staff called and prodded Tshepiso to hurry to the hospital from her town, a hundred kilometers to the north, and sign the necessary forms, she took her time. She arrived a week into Wabona's stay, barely greeted her husband, signed the required paper, and left immediately. It would have been easy enough to write her off as a lazy or selfish or callous woman. Perhaps the clinical staff thought so at the time. I don't know; I wasn't there. And what about this man's grown children, some of whom lived in Gaborone, yet failed to visit him? But the truth was that Wabona had spent the first fifteen years of his marriage beating Tshepiso senseless each time he came home from the bars in the evening, until she finally moved out. His children loathed him, as did his wife. Cancer did not change this. Instead, to them it felt almost like some form of justice.

If a crucial part of effective nursing is performing the proxy work of family, providing care in the context of moral sentiment, humanizing patients, marking the ward as a social and moral space, patients and their family members are critical actors, not passive recipients of these processes. Cancer renders patients vulnerable, it harms them, it hurts them, it worries them, and in this is a great equalizer. But American narratives of heroic survivors aside, cancer does not redeem patients, render them angelic, unless they began their path toward illness already so constituted. Nor does it undermine the deeply social nature of their personhood. Patients and relatives are fully human in ways both large and small, good and bad, complex and contradictory. They arrive in the cancer ward already embroiled in complex interactions, and these relationships spill into the clinical space, gathering nurses, doctors, and even fellow patients into their dynamics.

Social patterns, tensions, and values from beyond the clinic door continually seep into the ward, shaping its processes and patterns of care. Like so many hospitals, PMH is a tough and at times alienating institution—one with a dense bureaucracy and gritty facilities. Successful care therefore often hinges on the efforts of relatives to monitor the care of their patients, a job made more difficult by the highly regimented visiting hours. Some relatives finesse this by working alongside nurses or befriending them. Others complain to Dr. P or the hospital superintendent about the care received, and Dr. P might, in turn, take the nurses to task. Unlike the patterns documented in South Africa or Bangladesh, where middle-class nurses might look down on their poor patients, in Botswana nurses are in the middle of a class spectrum whose income differentials have expanded greatly in recent years, and this shapes the politics of patient advocacy.[33] Many nurses make a point of resisting claims that elite Batswana relatives make for extra resources (bed space, time with the doctor, nursing attention, rubber gloves to take home, etc.). Wealthy relatives are often more effective in advocating than are the relatives of poorer patients, so nurses might take on the role of advocate. Sometimes this may be because they are pushing back or bristling at what they consider the excessive demands of the wealthy, who they feel look on them as equivalent to maids. Other times it may be because they have sympathy for the plight of someone who is poor and who seems to ask so little of her caregivers, despite the depth of her needs.

But in many other cases, the therapy management group reconfigures in the ward into a powerful nurse-clinician-kin-neighbor hybrid, as relatives, doctors, and nurses work together to enact care for their patient. Relatives might go into the city or even across the border to

South Africa to purchase medicines or nursing supplies not available in the ward. Meanwhile, nurses might be enlisted by Dr. P to convince distant relatives to pursue a particular therapeutic strategy. With all these individuals operating in concert, care proceeds.

On Valentine's Day of 2007, at approximately three in the afternoon, the ambulance brought a group of six acute myeloid leukemia patients, all in their early twenties, back from South Africa, where they had been sent for treatment. One of them, a twenty-one-year-old man from Bobonong, tall, thin, and wearing a track suit, arrived with a fever and so was not discharged along with his friends. When Dr. P told him he could not continue on to his home, but instead would have to stay in PMH and potentially even return to South Africa, he was extremely upset. He was being left behind. "No, I just want to go home, I want to go back to school! I need to get back home." As he got angrier and quieter, Dr. P got angrier and louder, until finally he pounded his fist on the table and yelled, "NO, I ORDER YOU, as your doctor, to get into that ward!" Then Dr. P performed a pantomime of what would happen—shaking, convulsion—if the blood infection were to go untreated. Dr. P was furious that the patient had been sent from South Africa in this condition. The patient looked like he might cry as his friends slipped away toward their homes and he remained behind in PMH.

By the next morning, the young man was despondent during rounds, but his temperature was down. Then it turned out that, in a failed attempt to be discharged, he had been improperly placing the thermometer. He looked so depressed that Mma M, the ward matron, again counseled him extensively on how important it was to take care of the blood infection and assured him that he would be home before he knew it. I offered to give him my cell phone to call home, but he had in fact called a friend the day before. He told me that the problem was that there was no phone at home, so he could not speak with his family. This led to a longer conversation with Mma M, who took on an increasingly maternal tone, cajoling and counseling. And then, in the middle of their talk, in walked his mother, still smelling like the fire in the cooking enclosure back home.[34]

A few minutes later the surgeon arrived to remove the central intravenous line that was the most likely portal for the infection. But the patient refused the procedure. Mma M, the surgeon, the student nurse, and Dr. A all attempted to convince him to consent to the procedure. Dr. P arrived and insisted—demanded—that the procedure be done there and then. This pushed the patient a bit closer to passivity, but he was not there yet. And then his mother turned to him and said in Setswana, "I have come all the way from Bobonong to PMH. That is one hundred pula [bus fare], and I didn't come all this way to see you refuse [by which she meant die]." Then she and I laughed. I don't know why, but something about how she had referred to the bus fare was terrifically funny, and we both realized it at the same time. Her joking and her laughter were a way of saying that everything was going to be fine, that this was nothing serious — even though her visit showed how very serious it was, even as the laughter allowed tears to stream down her face. Dr. P was still saying, "Go home for what? Go home and this infection will kill you and you will die." But it no longer mattered. The patient was now busy requesting that his mother be allowed stay with him for the procedure. Sometimes mothers exceed the limits of even the most powerful of doctors and most effective of nurses.

CONCLUSION

Through its nurses, its patients, and its practices, the PMH oncology ward serves as a place where an ethic of social healing animates care-giving, offering powerful insights about the morality of care and the mutual dynamics of embodiment that shape care. Nurses and their patients do not always succeed in their efforts; a few have days where they appear to have even given up trying. And yet, day after day, patients arrive in PMH oncology. If they are not in deep bodily distress on arrival, they may well be on discharge. Such is the nature of healing via chemotherapy and radiation. The PMH cancer ward is a place where the stakes of moral sentiment and bodily care are high, where ailing human bodies provide the grounds on which politics and sociality are enacted in ways both large and small.

CODA: DEATH OF A VISITOR TO THE WARD

25 May 2009

When a patient from PMH oncology dies at home, relatives call the ward and tell the nurses, "Your patient has died." When the patient dies in the ward, the call goes in reverse.

During lunchtime, the woman in the ward in Female A Bed 2, who was paralyzed from the waist down, with a possible developing pressure sore—this older woman—died. Mma O discovers the death and pulls the curtain around her bed. I go to help Mma O and Mma J to process her body. Mma H comes in and says, "Ao! She didn't even wait to see her kids. Me, I want to die at home." Mma J says, "Yes, I also want to die that side." We all agree that we do. Mma O rolls her (a big woman, about sixty years old) to the side so that Mma J can remove the catheter. I help to hold her on her side. First they inject some water so that the balloon can be pulled out. Then Mma H spreads her [the patient's] legs, and Mma O pulls it [the catheter] out. She [the patient] is all splayed, genitals showing (though of course the curtain is closed tight), and smelling rotten. Now Mma J will work to restore order to her body. Even a dead body can be humanized, must be humanized. Using cotton wool and alcohol, they wipe away the bits of feces clinging in her anus, and whatever else is smelling. They remove the cannulas. Then (we are all wearing gloves and plastic aprons) we put her legs lying straight and closed, her arms fixed to her sides, placing her fingers under her buttocks and hips to hold the arms in place. This takes some strength and determination. Mma J takes the top blanket and smooths it and folds it and then uses it as a pillow to put her head in place. She is looking more like a funeral corpse now. Then Mma J keeps trying to close her mouth. It keeps gaping, and so she wraps it with a bandage from chin to the top of her head to set it in place as she stiffens. We pull up the blankets to her chin, making sure they cover her feet. Then we pack her belongings into two black garbage bags. This whole process has taken some muscle, some care, and some respect.

While all of this is going on, Dr. Z is poring over her files, trying to figure out what happened. This woman had been in female ortho, but then came to oncology within the last few days. Was I there for the transfer? She was from Tsabong [a town in the Kalahari], but didn't get to go back and "die that side" because the transport last Friday only had an FWE [a village health worker] and she needed to travel with a nurse.

I walk into the clinic office, and Dr. R says, "Hey! I find it so, so sad. Her family, her children back in Tsabong. Just saying to themselves, 'I hope everything in PMH is going well'—and to die so far from home without anyone to talk to . . ."

FIVE

Pain and Laughter

The PMH oncology ward is brimming with pain. Patients sit gripping their chairs in the clinic office as metastases burrow into their clavicles. They shuffle down the hallway, doubled over from a pelvis packed with tumor. The ward holds an array of instruments of torture: the boring needle for the bone-marrow biopsy, the flexible nasogastric tubes which are rammed up the noses and down the throats of those who can barely swallow, the van to the radiation machine, from which some patients emerge scorched black, as if they have crawled out of a smoldering fire, their mouths packed with sores. At the same time, the PMH oncology ward is also absolutely hilarious. Nurses trade mock insults with Dr. P, patients crack jokes and laugh at the images of their own deaths, nursing assistants and patients giggle at Dr. P's attempts at Setswana. Rarely have I worked in a place where I laughed as hard as I did in the PMH oncology ward. The laughter and the pain are often conjoined here, though the ward is marked by a general absence of Schadenfreude.

In what follows I look closely at some of the more fine-grained processes of clinical care to suggest how cancer, as an emergent issue in African public health, forces long-standing questions of palliation to the foreground, highlighting the intensely social nature of pain. Cancer and palliative care share a history, and pain highlights the particular somatic predicament of Africa's cancer patients. I contemplate the conditions that facilitate the marginalization of pain and palliation in African clinical practice and global health more widely. As Human Rights Watch has documented, though cancer rates are rising, widespread shortages and in many cases the outright absence of strong pain relief are the norm across much of the global south.[1] I examine the contemporary clinical dynamics this engenders in a specific context—oncology, where many patients have severe intractable pain, and where others are grappling with the painful effects of biomedical therapies. In other words, the ward offers an opportunity to explore how and why biomedicine proceeds in Africa with so little palliation and so much compliance. I provide brief histories of the local poetics of endurance, and of race and pain in biomedicine that are necessary to understand these dynamics. Importantly, the ward also offers a place to consider how palliation operates, how pain is communicated, witnessed, and imbued with meaning. Many of Botswana's cancer patients have aggressive and advanced disease. Such cancers are often relentlessly painful, and clinicians may respond to them with therapies that are deeply aversive.[2] At the same time, because such patients are understood to be very sick, and because many of them become known to clinical staff through cyclical visits and hospitalizations, the ethic of palliation that holds in the ward is unique in the hospital and the broader health system.[3]

In highlighting the social nature of pain, I join those who question Elaine Scarry's now famous proposition that pain is an individually held experience, one that "shatters language."[4] Scarry found that pain simultaneously produces certainty in the person in pain and doubt in the onlooker, a dynamic of witnessing (and even of inflicting) from which cascade a series of ethical problems around what to do about pain. She goes on to examine these ethical problems of *doing*, in part through an examination of texts on torture, war, scripture, memoir, and Marx, all the while rendering pain as an object located in an individually bounded body. Yet this conceptualization is ill suited to capture the logics of pain and the processes of palliation in Botswana's oncology ward, and, I suspect, in many other places. Moreover, textual analysis is perhaps too thin a base from which to make sense of these complex forms of experience and communication. Ethnography offers competing perspectives.

In my conversations with Tswana healers, I found that it was nearly impossible to talk about pain as pain, to imbue it with ontological import, to construct it as an object. Pain, it seemed, could not be separated out; it collapsed back into its underlying pathology, which in Tswana medicine is necessarily a social pathology.[5] This total situatedness of pain, its refusal to be separated from the flow of pathological social experience is meaningful, and it helps us move from the problem that doubt presents to the social effects of certainty.[6]

The oncology ward is an intensely social space, one where doubt is simply not at the center of the problem of doing that pain presents. Everyone knows with certainty that drilling into a patient's bone marrow or sawing off a patient's leg produces pain, yet this pain is engendered to heal, even as it might be ignored. In this social approach to pain, I am in sympathy with the anthropologist Talal Asad's ideas about the body, agency, and pain, which contrast with Scarry's proposition. In moving from text to experience, from the specificity of torture to broader categories of social interaction, Asad does not see pain as an object to be overcome by an agentive individual. Instead, he argues, pain is a relationship. Asad acknowledges that somatic experiences of injured persons cannot be fully accessed by observers, but he reminds us that that is not all pain is. He writes, "Sufferers are also social persons (animals) and their suffering is partly constituted by the way they inhabit, or are constrained to inhabit, their relationship with others."[7] In other words, pain begs a response. Sometimes that response is laughter. To open up the social dynamics of pain and palliation, I offer, unfortunately, a somewhat grisly excerpt from my ethnographic field notes.

AFTER THE AMPUTATION

25 January 2007

A Kaposi's sarcoma patient, M. This man is in his thirties—he was amputated above the knee on the 15th. We are on ward rounds, visiting cancer patients in men's surgical, and he requests to see Dr. P. Dr. P asks for him to be brought to the oncology clinic after rounds. I remember the meeting before the amputation, and how M willingly agreed to rid himself of the swollen, rotting, and now useless leg. It was thick like a tree trunk, the skin rough like bark, and it sounded hollow when thumped. Later in the morning, M arrives in oncology from the men's surgical ward in a wheelchair with an orderly. He is in CRAZY pain. His eyes are bulging and rolling, and he is pouring sweat. He is in agony. [I looked later at his medical card. He was originally given pethidine, 100 mgs, then tapering to 50 mgs, then codeine for a few days, then, for about a week preceding this encounter, ibuprofen only.][8] He is anxious, and he tells Dr. P, "They want to push me out—to send me home! But I can't manage. There is a problem with the leg. You can even smell it." Dr. P tries to touch up high on the stump, and M cringes in agony. Silent, but in agony nonetheless. I am on the edge of my seat, cringing, and wondering if I should say something about the obvious pain. Dr. P seems cognizant of the pain, but not particularly interested in it. Intense. At one point, he absently places his hand on M's thigh as a sign of compassion, and M recoils with force. Dr. P has him unwind the bandage and show the wound. M is squirming in pain as he does it, and as he gets down to the last layer of gauze he is really crying out short breathy sounds. Eesh! Tjo Tjo Tjo! With force. It is unbearable, and it is just coming out of his mouth involuntarily. M speaks excellent English. Then, as he gets to the point of exposing the wound, it is too much and he can't go on. I fear he will pass out. I can see that Dr. P is a bit impatient, and I know why. There is a tremendous queue of patients waiting for him (the only oncologist), many of them are very ill, and this is taking a long time. Besides, it is a surgical problem, not the KS that is causing this.

So Dr. P calls for a nurse, and Mma L comes. Dr. P asks her to take M to the treatment room across the hall and take off the bandage with water, it is stuck to the wound. "And please give 75 mgs pethidine first. As you can see, it is very painful." Mma L glances over at M and protests that she is covering the ward and she can't also be here. Dr. P says, "Where is Mma M, who should be here?" Mma M has gone on tea break. A little debate, and then Mma L agrees to do it. But she wants Dr. P to put the pethidine order on the hospital card. He says he will do it later. "No, you must do it first." All the while, I am squirming, feeling like I am the only one with a sense of urgency about the pain here. I also feel like M must be so freaked out to see his leg like this. He is only ten days after the surgery. Who knows how he is currently making sense of the trauma of profound disfigurement?

We leave and go to the private ward to see another patient. When we return, Dr. P is about to eat a peach for his impromptu tea when Mma T says, "No, don't eat that. You need to go and look at the leg in the treatment room first." "What? It will make me vomit—I won't want to eat afterwards." So we have some joking. Dr. P quickly finishes his peach and washes his hands.

We enter the treatment room, and M's stump is covered with a piece of gauze just resting on it. M is still sweating, and his eyes are still bulging, but he is calmer after the pethidine. Dr. P lifts the gauze and exposes the wound—it has completely burst the sutures. The jagged end of the bone is jutting out like a roast beef, and it is all totally infected, swollen, white rot-

ting meat. They failed to disarticulate the bone during the surgery.[9] He can't possibly be discharged. Nor should he be transferred to oncology—he needs to be re-amputated immediately. And as Dr. A says, the remainder of the femur [must be] removed and the wound closed. I am appalled. Dr. P less so. Dr. A comes in and is a bit dazed by it, asking if we've seen it (Did he say it? Or did he say, "The guy with the KS amputation"? Or did he say, "M"?), and then commenting on how dangerous this is. I remember this patient— I remember M—he had accepted the need for amputation and was almost cheerful about it—now this. If I were his relative, I would be through the roof. Go ferosa sebete.

THE POLITICS OF PAIN RELIEF

My purpose in presenting this visceral example is not to exploit M for theatrical purposes, and I confess that I feel a bit uncomfortable about exposing the intimacies of his vulnerability. Yet, given how abstract (and in doubt) the pain of others can be, I fear that ethnography of this sort is necessary in order to ask you to imagine being in extreme and serious bodily distress, groping for some sort of communicative possibility that will bring relief to you, in an institutional setting where the mechanisms of relief are closely controlled, and where the nearest thing to a relative or friend you might have—someone actually invested in you—is, you are hoping, this German oncologist.[10] At the same time, I am asking you to imagine being a nurse or a doctor in a chronically overwhelmed hospital, a decade into an AIDS epidemic in which you have seen so much suffering and death.

What are we to make of this decidedly African scene, with its German oncologist, Dr. P, and its profoundly overcrowded urban hospital named for a European princess? Setting aside the clinical issues of how this amputation went so wrong, we are left with the pain. Where were the pain charts of smiling and frowning faces, and the 1–5 pain scales of contemporary American and European hospitals?[11] How could someone in such obvious distress not have been given pain medicine sooner? Why did M draw attention to the smell of his leg, but not complain of his substantial pain? Why did I (and perhaps you) feel such discomfort at M's obvious pain, and the clinical staff less so, even though Dr. P and the oncology nurses were caring people and passionate about their work? How and why did M manage to stay so relatively calm and quiet in the face of such agony? Why does almost every patient seem to leave the hospital or clinic with a packet of paracetamol or ibuprofen—whether they need it or not—yet many clinical staff are reluctant to use opioids even for patients who are dying, despite long-standing WHO protocols encouraging their use? How could we be joking and laughing about this human leg of rotting meat while enjoying a peach?

It is ironic that biomedicine proceeds in Africa with so little palliation, given that pain is what propels many patients into clinics and (often iatrogenic) hospital spaces. Health planners go through great effort to get patients to come to biomedical sites, rather than consult "traditional" healers, yet they seem generally, albeit with some exceptions, to ignore this fundamental bodily experience as motivation. The sheer force of pain has many swimming upstream in an overwrought health system. True, there is now an African palliative-care movement, but so much has been pushed under this rubric, from the writing of wills to the provision of basic nutrition, that the imperative of pain itself has been diluted.[12] The fact of pain, the desire for relief, and the phenomenology and materiality of palliation are not to be underestimated, even though much of it seems to happen around the edges and in the interstitial spaces of African healthcare.

In Botswana there is a particular economy of expression and an ethic of palliation, such that pain may be spoken of, but rarely screamed or cried over, and this has critical effects in contemporary clinical practice, as does a nursing culture that has historically shied away from the use of strong painkillers.[13] But we should not romanticize patient silence. A national survey of terminally ill patients and their caregivers conducted in four districts of the country found that 64 percent of respondents listed "severe pain" as a crucial problem of the terminally ill, making it the most commonly reported issue.[14] Nor is the problem limited to Botswana. Another study that contrasted the experience of dying of cancer in Scotland and western Kenya found that "the emotional pain of facing death was the primary concern of Scottish patients and their carers, while physical pain and financial worries dominated the lives of Kenyan patients and their carers."[15]

Though pharmaceutical interventions are only one aspect of pain relief, and their introduction into places like Botswana does not occur in a vacuum, they are nonetheless suggestive of the wider problem. In 2004 the International Narcotics Control Board reported, "Developing countries, which represent about 80 per cent of the world's population, accounted for only about 6 per cent of global consumption of morphine."[16] The statistics are telling. For example, in 2007 Botswana (with its AIDS and cancer epidemics, and all the attendant pain that implies) consumed an estimated 1.58 milligrams of therapeutic morphine equivalents per person.[17] My educated guess is that much of this consumption occurred in the country's cancer ward. Compare that figure to that of the United States, where consumption was 648 milligrams per capita.[18]

The problems are complex. Maintaining adequate stocks of drugs (any drugs) in African health systems has long been problematic. Even when adequate national stocks of morphine are available, they are difficult for many nonhospitalized patients to access, due to barriers of travel, the need for professional referral from clinic to hospital, and other logistical and economic considerations.[19] There is reluctance to allow nurses to prescribe opiates, although it is nurses who by and large staff rural health centers. This is certainly the case in Botswana, where opioids are available only in the pharmacies of referral hospitals, and where morphine or codeine regularly go in and out of stock (as do all medical supplies). And the presence of opioids in a broader pharmacy network could promote the development of a black market in highly addictive drugs — a dynamic the ministry of health quite understandably wishes to avoid. In addition, the lack of expectation around chemical palliation also shapes patient demands. In other words, if patients do not expect that such relief is possible, then they are much less likely to demand it. But these problems of access are not directly related to price in the ways we have seen for Gleevec or many other cancer drugs, or for antiretrovirals in the 1990s. Morphine, codeine, and pethidine are all easily available for low cost from the generics industry. That "the world's twenty richest countries consume 80% of global therapeutic morphine" is a fact created out of a complex political, economic, technocratic, and cultural history.

Until the past decade or so, the kinds of statistics I just presented were aggregated by the narcotics board but not discussed in public health outside of the domains of global cancer and palliative care. For many years, other issues have seemed more pressing in the zero-sum world of global health, where various diseases and tools compete for attention and resources. And laws and policies governing the distribution of opiates have been far more concerned with halting drug abuse and trafficking (admittedly important problems) than with the other use of opiates—

pain relief. Fortunately, due to the hard work of many activists, a global palliative-care movement is under way, and in a very few select places this situation has begun (but only just begun) to change.

But how could institutions charged with promoting health and providing care have ignored a phenomenon as fundamental as pain for so long? From a policy and planning perspective, it makes some sense. Most health systems in the global south historically have been evaluated through a system of metrics that measures the transmission of infectious disease, mortality, live births, life expectancy, and other qualitative measures. In this macrosystem of evaluation, the experience of illness is rendered invisible. Pain management becomes something of a frill—distracting from the core concerns of healthcare. And if pain relief isn't available, and if doctors and nurses are not trained to prioritize it, then patients don't expect to receive it. They don't ask for it, relatives don't demand it, and so pain remains depoliticized in healthcare, even as patients writhe in agony. In this context, pain management can seem a luxury, rather than an imperative in policy formulations, and this also manifests itself in the daily logics of clinical practice.

In a place where the reliance on chemical analgesics is greatly attenuated, as it is in Botswana, efforts to socialize pain are particularly important, if subtle. Nowhere, perhaps, is this more important than in relation to cancer. In the colposcopy clinic, the gynecologist Dr. T diagnoses cervical cancers. He remarks to me that the women here endure pain *much* differently than do women in Europe—even for stage 3 cervical cancer. He says he has to struggle to convince the nurses to administer morphine, because the patients will tolerate the pain with just ibuprofen. In 1994, a survey in Botswana asked sixty-five nurses to identify their standard analgesic drug of choice for treatment of "severe pain." The results were typical of those reported in other parts of the global south: over a third chose paracetamol (Tylenol); another 23 percent chose Panado (Tylenol) with codeine; 16.9 percent chose 50 mgs of pethidine (Demerol); and the remaining 20 percent chose 75 mgs of pethidine. In the same study, the researcher created hypothetical patient scenarios. She found that "a shocking 23 percent would not even give morphine" to a grimacing post-abdominal-surgery patient who reported a 4 on a 1–5 pain scale, and who had a doctor's order in his chart for 5–15 mgs of morphine PRN (as needed), 4 hourly.[20]

In the cancer ward, there is less hesitation to palliate chemically. Dr. P jokes that he beat it out of the nurses when he arrived, this reluctance to use strong painkillers. This is a good joke: pain is inflicted on some to ameliorate it in others. Hospitals are full of such jokes, and in Botswana there is a rich tradition of joking about beating. Nurses in oncology do take note of pain and will advocate on behalf of patients for relief when they think it necessary.[21]

Oncology in particular is a set of grueling and at times brutal and violent practices, albeit ones performed with great hope and determination. And cancers themselves are often extremely and relentlessly painful in their own right. And yet clinical oncology, like all public biomedical care in Botswana, proceeds with few of the niceties — the powerful anti-emetics, the morphine pumps, the fentanyl patches, the sedatives, the informational literature, the counseling — meant to smooth the rough edges of chemotherapy, radiation burns, severe mucositis, surgical wounds, nasogastric tubes, and invasive diagnostic procedures.

Surely cost has something to do with this utilitarian approach to healthcare. But morphine and codeine are inexpensive drugs. Cost alone cannot explain how a health system can afford to administer complex chemotherapy to a lymphoma patient but not properly palliate a terminally ill woman whose radiation treatments for her cervical cancer have created an inoperable fistula so deep and painful that she tries by all measures to resist her own hunger — so intense is her fear of the pain of defecation.

STRIVING FOR SILENCE

Most patients comply with painful diagnostic and therapeutic procedures with minimal complaint. Some patients, of course, simply fail to return for subsequent rounds of dreaded chemotherapy, and others reach a point in the advancement of metastatic disease and treatment complications where they are so overwhelmed by the pain that they cry out or grip the nurse's (or visiting ethnographer's) arm in a silent plea for help. Over time, in moments of acute, yet enduring agony, pain has the ability to grind down the resolve of even those highly practiced in the art of forbearance, such that eventually even the scratch of the sheets, the prick of the needle, and the grip of the blood-pressure cuff become exquisite insults. Many do not mention their pain unless directly asked about it by the doctor, nurse, or ethnographer, but when asked what the problem is, such patients will readily report pain, with great firmness.

This is not to say that there is no complaint. After exchanging greetings during social visits and clinical encounters alike, elderly women often recite a litany of places where their bodies hurt. Such are the privileges of old age. And in many ways the minor insult is easier to express than the major one. In the 1970s and 1980s, some doctors described what they assumed was a somaticization of emotional stress, in the form of sore throats, headaches, or generalized body pains.[22] Patients or relatives sometimes protest the nausea of chemotherapy, which for some patients can be overwhelming. Others express anger at having been "burned by the machine" during radiotherapy, especially if it failed to cure. Nor does their silent endurance of pain mean that patients do not want material assistance. A gynecologist once joked with a nurse and me in the colposcopy clinic that we should just put out a big bowl of ibuprofen, like Smarties (candy). It is really all that patients want, even as Batswana friends and acquaintances often expressed cynicism about how ibuprofen and paracetamol were dispensed in lieu of care. But generally, in Botswana, people from approximately age five and up are expected to undergo all but the worst pain in silence. The few who do cry "excessively" are sources of utter hilarity for both onlookers (including medical staff) and themselves. This means that subtle calculations are continually made by onlookers, who would never laugh at the cries of a patient they deemed to be in true agony or distress.

The poetics of pain, and the malleability, the slipperiness, the diversity of this foundational human experience and mode of expression underscore the importance of what the anthropologist Margaret Lock has famously termed "local biology." This concept argues against the universal human body posited by biomedicine, by suggesting instead that "biological difference—sometimes obvious, at other times very subtle—molds and contains the subjective experience of individuals and the creation of cultural interpretations."[23] The historical ecology of care (including the availability of analgesics), of bodily practice, of diet, disease, and other such factors shape experiences of pain by situating bodies, emplotting them in particular histories.[24]

SILENCE IN BLACK, BROWN, AND WHITE

18 June 2008
Achieving Silence in the Surgical Ward

We are rounding in female surgical ward, because we don't have a bed in oncology for Margaret, the woman with the massive Burkitt's lymphoma swelling in her thigh. While there, we can visit our postmastectomy patients. At the far end of the cubicle, I see Dr. S, a senior surgeon from India who's been working at PMH for decades, with his team. The woman in bed 1 begins crying out in pain as he palpates her. We all turn to look. Dr. S is firm and a bit irritated. "No, mma, you may not do that! We see these problems all the time, and I know it may hurt, but it is no reason to cry." He chastises her further and then continues with his exam. She is now quiet, with maybe seven or eight people all looking at her.

31 March 2007
Almost Achieving Silence in the Obstetrics
and Gynecology Ward

9:30 PM. I arrive at the Labor department for the night shift, and meet Dr. M, a Bangladeshi doctor in his early forties, who is currently assigned to Obs and Gynae. We go straight to Gynae. There is a patient—a woman age forty-one—moaning and writhing in pain. She is in the corridor on a narrow gurney. She has had pethidine in Accident and Emergency and is still in a good deal of pain. Dr. M takes her case history. She's been bleeding and gets bad pain each period since 2001, but this time is by far the worse. Grava 5 para 2 [five pregnancies, two viable deliveries]. Dr. M examines, and suspects fibroids—he can feel a large one. As he examines and she cries out, he says each time firmly, but gently, "No. Try to tolerate." And she does. The crying stops, but she is still moaning. An obese woman in bra and panty. She's had 80 mgs pethidine already, but when we see her she is still writhing, putting her leg into the handle of the supply closet door to brace herself while on the exam table, clutching the table, and so on. Dr. M tells the nurse to give her 100 mg IM stat of pethidine. It is amazing that she was in so much pain, but when she had to climb from the stretcher onto the exam table, she just was able to focus and get it done, though I am sure it was a huge challenge for her. Dr. M. explains to her that this is very painful, but not life-threatening. But that it will have to come out.

31 January 2007
Achieving Silence during a Bone-Marrow
Biopsy in Oncology

*It is about 4:30 PM, nearing the end of a long day that began at 7:45 AM
in the incredible heat of Botswana's summer. This will be Dr. A's very first
bone-marrow biopsy. He has watched Dr. P perform many of these procedures—but now it is his turn to try himself. The patient, O, speaks good English. He has been waiting on one of the long benches outside the clinic for
his turn. O is in his mid-forties, and he has what looks like a hematological
tumor in his abdomen, of unknown origin. By sampling his bone marrow,
Dr. P hopes to identify the precise nature of the tumor and to learn if the
tumor is a metastasis that actually originated in O's bone marrow. This is
explained to O: "We are to do a test so that we can help you with your cancer. You will need to lie still."*

*Mma H, one of the nursing sisters (a really excellent nurse), in her early
thirties, sets up a sterile surgical pack on the small cart next to the high, narrow exam table. We pull the exam table away from the wall so that Dr. P
can fit alongside Dr. A, a medical officer [a resident, in American terms] from
Egypt who has been assigned to the oncology ward, though his specialty is
actually anesthesia. Mma H, a student nurse, and I are all on the other side.
After being instructed to do so, O takes his shoes off, pulls his trousers off,
folds them and places them on an empty chair, pulls up his T-shirt a bit, to
expose his buttocks. He lies face down, head tilted toward Mma H and I on
the table, the student a bit behind us. "You must remain still." Drs. P and A
both put on sterile gloves from the packs over the regular latex exam gloves.*

*Dr. A wipes the area with betadine [a rust-colored antiseptic]. They give O
a shot of local anesthetic first. This will numb the flesh on his buttock and
make it possible for them to go through the flesh with the big boring needle.
But it will not numb the bone itself. The needle is very large, and hollow.
O is lying on his stomach and so he cannot see how big the needle is. Dr. A
guides it in until he hits the bone, then he pulls the needle guide out. "Now
comes the painful part. The anesthetic we use does nothing for the pain of
extraction," Dr. P explains to me, knowing my interest in pain. "Keep still,"
they tell O, and I keep my hand on O's upper back in what I hope is a gesture of comfort and solidarity. Dr. A starts drilling into the bone, twisting
the boring needle in a mechanical way that requires deep pressure and hard
physical labor. Turning and turning the needle with effort. At one point,
Dr. P has to step in, because Dr. A is not hitting the bone quickly enough.*

He lays his hands over Dr. A's and guides him, showing him how the bone runs in one direction and it will be easier to run with the bone. O's eyes are open. He is still. Dr. A keeps drilling. Dr. P explains to me, "You see, as you drill in, it pushes the material further in, so in extracting the sample you have to wiggle the drill back out while holding a finger over the opening in the needle where you removed the guide—this will make a vacuum." It has been at least fifteen minutes. Mma H turns to me and says, "Botlhoko!" [Setswana for pain]. This is one of the first times I have seen a nurse really comment on the pain of a procedure so explicitly [though certainly when I have watched and assisted nurses cleaning necrotic wounds, I have observed that they are intensely aware of and sensitive to the pain]. I almost don't dare look at poor O—but there he is, still as can be, his face pouring sweat. My only job was to open the specimen container of formalin and pour a bit out to make room for the sample, and even this small thing I was having a hard time managing. The last thing I wanted was to be the reason this procedure needed to be repeated.

Dr. A pulls out the core sample and drops slices of it into my jar of formalin. He, too, is sweating. Dr. P puts the lid on the container and then, not trusting the pathologist entirely, presses a few pieces between glass slides to examine personally, taking care not to crush the cells. Dr. A presses a piece of betadine-soaked gauze over the wound, and then we hand him strips of tape to cover it. He and Dr. P pull off their gloves and step out of the clinic and across the breezeway to the lab to take the slides for staining. Mma H folds up the used surgical packs and goes with the student nurse to deposit the used instruments.

O pulls up his trousers, and comes and sits down next to me on one of the other empty chairs in the clinic room. He turns to me and quite calmly says in a combination of Setswana and English, "Well, that was certainly the worst pain I have ever experienced in my life. Please tell me that they don't ever do that to children. I can't even imagine what would happen if they did that to a child." He looks a bit dazed. I say, "OK, I won't tell you, but, yes, it is done to children, and it takes several adults holding them down to accomplish." "Tell me again, why exactly they did that to me?" I try to give him a more detailed explanation of the biomedical logic behind the procedure. It is hard to express in Setswana, and I stick mostly to English. But I, too, am dazed. Even though Mma H had said, "Botlhoko!" I hadn't fully realized the extent, I think, since O had lain there so calmly, until I talked to him afterward. O wants to leave to catch his bus, he needs to squeeze into a crowded

*minibus taxi to the bus rank, from which he will catch a bumpy bus ride to
a stop in his village, and then walk the path to his house. I check with the
doctors and let O go. He will return next week for the results.*[25]

8 January 2007
Silence Achieved but Not Assumed:
The Bone Marrow Aspirate

*Mr. J, about sixty years old, arrives at Accident and Emergency. It looks like
he may have leukemia, and so Dr. P is called from oncology. The patient
has been referred from the primary hospital at Ramotswa. Dr. P, Dr. A,
and I walk to Accident and Emergency, where we are shown to the second
cubicle. We go behind the curtain and lying there is a white man, big and
burly, in knee socks and khaki shorts and shirt. He must be South African.
Boer? Dr. P encourages him to return to South Africa to get his care. "No,
Doc. I am a Motswana. Ke tswa Lobatse." "Do you have insurance? We
can send you to the private hospital or to South Africa." No. His daughter is
there, and she shows us his Omang [national identity] card. It is unusual to
have a white patient in the public hospital, but by no means unprecedented.
And at times there have been more than one white patient in the oncology
queue or lying in the ward. He will be admitted. But first Dr. P wants to do
a bone-marrow aspirate on the spot, to confirm his suspected diagnosis so
that treatment can begin. He pushes the needle hard into the sternum with
force, boring into the bone, but when he pulls up the plunger there is no
fluid. A dry aspirate—he must try again. Mr. J grimaces, but remains silent.
But Dr. A reaches over and holds his hand, and his daughter holds the other
one. The Motswana nurse comforts him with gentle words and strokes his
forehead. I try to imagine this happening to* monna mogolo. *His whiteness
apparently creates different expectations around his stoicism. Another dry
tap. The third time the extraction works. Mr J is quiet and calm, but after it
is finished he manages a smile.*

Over the course of Mr. J's care, which, sadly, lasted only a few months
before he died, he spent many days in the oncology ward and had many
visits to the oncology clinic. He was fluent in Setswana and quite good-
natured. He, his wife, his adult children, and his parents and grandparents had spent all of their lives in Botswana. At one point, I was surprised,
because of their apparent racial difference, to learn that he was the half-
uncle of another Motswana patient in the ward. In many ways he was
as much a Motswana as O was, and they both had leukemia (though of

different types), yet Mr. J had doctors and nurses holding his hands, re-assuring him with words and explaining procedures, while M heard only Mma H's "Botlhoko!" In southern Africa there is a long history of per-forming subtle, racialized differences of pain experience. Such perfor-mances find their origins, in part, in a longer history of race, pain, and medicine.

SILENCE AS HISTORY

Earlier British and American observers were fascinated by the pain of Africans, noting their forbearance. They channeled this fascination into three related assumptions: first, that Africans actually feel less pain than their white counterparts; second, that Africans are more stoic than whites and thus bear their pain more calmly; and third, unlike the cult of sensitivity and empathy that distinguishes bourgeois British sensibili-ties, that Africans possess a certain callousness with regard to the suffer-ing of their fellow human beings. Over time, these ideas were articulated in terms less sentimental and more scientific, until they just became a sort of common sense. It is quite likely (though somewhat more diffi-cult to document) that Africans held inverse assumptions, both about the hypersensitivity of Europeans and their overwrought pain perfor-mances. Certainly, such ideas are evident today in Botswana, as when women broke into utter hilarity when discussing with me the foolishness of white women's moaning and screaming during labor—the humor only compounded by the image of these white women bringing their men into the delivery room![26] All these debates, all these ghosts mingle in Botswana's central hospital. It is a place where European, South and East Asian, North American, Cuban, and African staff merge, interact, and circulate to create a clinical culture, one in which African pain is mar-veled at, pitied, and outright ignored in ways that both stun and dull the visiting American observer.

There is no direct historical arrow that links today's hospital with yesterday's British missionary or travel writer, no unbroken narrative that can connect the cancer patient awaiting a bone-marrow biopsy or reamputation with the men whose fibrous tumors David Livingstone re-moved with a knife in his crudely erected shelter in the veldt, all the while admiring their forbearance.[27] But there are continuities worth contem-plating, ideas and practices that have sedimented into embodied life and which may help explain why until quite recently questions of pain relief were all but ignored in African biomedicine. The point is not that African hospital staff are callous and other non-African staff are not callous (though visiting American clinical staff often imply as much), but rather that all staff, regardless of race and national origin, seem to perceive and respond to patients' pain in ways that subtly acknowledge the patient's race.

In the late eighteenth century, as Karen Haltunnen explains, a British culture of humanitarian reform began to remake pain as a problem, an obscene one at that. Whereas previously pain had been understood to be an inevitable part of life, by the late eighteenth century, sentimentalism, and new ideas about empathy, had reconstructed pain as a moral crisis. Flogging, torture, and the physical punishments inflicted on slaves and asylum inmates were all problematized as uncivilized with the potential to morally debase and desensitize onlookers and victims alike.[28] This transition was as vital to and caught up in the development of anesthesia as it was to the abolition movement and the civilizing mission in southern Africa and beyond, and the shift from the spectacle of punishment to the regime of discipline that interested Michel Foucault. Pain became a new kind of (titillating) spectacle, a problem that inspired action.

By the mid-nineteenth century in the United States, which in some very broad sense shared a medical culture with Britain, "a new social awareness of, and sensitivity to, suffering helped shape such disparate movements as antislavery and antivivisection. Looking back on this era, philosopher Charles Pierce reportedly proposed that the nineteenth century be remembered as the 'Age of Pain.' Accompanying this change in social values, mid-century physicians experienced a technical revolution in the treatment of pain: the isolation of morphine, cocaine, and heroin; the invention of the hypodermic syringe, and, most dramatically, the discovery of inhalation anesthesia."[29] Yet, somehow, in the years that followed, the inhalation anesthesia crossed the south Atlantic without the morphine in tow.

Perhaps this was at least in part because pain had also long been a part of how people came to racialize one another and to judge one another's humanity, and thus action was often parsed along racial lines.[30] Racial ideas about pain facilitated the trade in African slaves, the colonial management of black and brown subjects throughout the British empire, and the development of medical knowledge (gynecology being the most infamous example).[31] Even as pain was problematized through a new ethos of humanitarian reform, and palliated through a set of chemicals that appeared to affect all people, regardless of race, these developments were still subordinated to older, persistent ideas about racial sensibilities.

British missionaries who arrived in Bechuanaland beginning in the early nineteenth century, like European and American travelers throughout Africa, embodied this contradictory sensibility, quite literally. Their writings are replete with descriptions of and references to their own physical pain, born of the indignities of the Africa environment with its (literally) blistering sun, clouds of stinging insects, accidents, animal bites, and fevers.[32] Phyllis Mack explains how for Methodist women in Britain, some of whom would arrive as early missionaries to the Batswana, pain, and bodily suffering more generally, presented *the* test of self-mastery that lay at the heart of an emergent female Methodist selfhood during this time. In other words, pain offered the potential for spiritual agency through suffering.[33] Evidence of the self-mastery Mack describes, both male and female, lay somewhere at the heart of the civilizing mission. These writers juxtaposed vivid descriptions of European pain to dulled African senses.

A typical example is provided by Mr. Thomson, a late-nineteenth-century British traveler in East Africa, who tells us of poor Mr. Johnston: "For a fortnight we carried him through swamps, and along great stretches of scrubby desert, in horrible pain from the disease, the jolting of the porters, and the intense heat of the tropical sun."[34] We can expect that the "we" who carried him may not have included Mr. Thomson himself. And yet the porters, whose jostling upset Mr. Johnston so, were not accorded the possibility of pain or heat as they moved with their load. Pain also provided, as it had during slavery, a way to enact these labor hierarchies without compromising the masculinity of whites. "The natives excel in carrying weights," we are told by a British observer, "which the civilized man drops through pain, not through weight; a hammock carried on a pole over the shoulder soon becomes unbearable to us if no pad be used, through the cutting into the shoulder, not from the weight itself; were the load more comfortably distributed we might carry it as easily as the native; it is insensibility to pain, not extra strength, that enables the native to bear such loads with ease."[35]

Hypotheses as to why Africans were so inured to pain ran a range. Harriet Roche, a British woman who traveled through southern Africa, attributed it to, of all things, the wondrous properties of a diet of early colonial impoverishment.

> It is astonishing how quickly a Kaffir gets over any injury, and how un-flinchingly he bears any surgical operation when he knows it is for his own good. I was told in Maritzburg, of one whose heel had been crushed by the falling of stone in some quarry the bone was cut away and a sil-ver plate put in. ("The beggar will run away with it if I don't keep my eye upon him," said the doctor who operated on him.) He *walked* off after all was over, and was well within a month. Much of this may be attrib-uted to the simple diet and habits of the native of South Africa. Noth-ing but mealy meal porridge from year's end to year's end. Meat he so rarely tastes that it almost intoxicates, so potent a food does it become when thus seldom eaten and then with such avidity and in such incred-ibly large quantities that the result is hardly to be wondered at. This meal, from the Indian corn grounded must have great life-restoring properties when men of such caliber as this "noble savage" are nourished into man-hood by it.[36]

J. G. Wood, a British author of several popular illustrated books on animals, aggregated a wide array of travelers' accounts from across the globe in his volume *The Uncivilized Races of Men in All Countries of the World*. Throughout his chronicling of various "races" of Africans, there is an insistent theme of insensitivity to pain. Hottentots, we learn, "suffer very little pain from injuries that would nearly kill a white man, or at all events would cause him to be nearly dead with pain alone."[37] While the Bushman's "hide was so tough that your arms would ache long before you produced any keen sense of pain by thrashing him."[38] Pain was pos-sible, but remote, given "the blunt nerves of an African."[39]

Of course there were contradictions. Europeans, particularly British missionaries, sometimes denied the existence of African pain, and at other times exhibited that same pain to suggest African callousness. No-where for missionaries was this pathological African apathy, this contrast between European (Christian) sensitivity and compassion and African insensitivity, more evident than in laughter. British observers found Afri-can laughter in the face of pain at best bewildering and at worst abhor-rent, as did Elizabeth Lees Price, who recorded the following in her Be-chuanaland journal in 1862.

Never should I forget the sight I beheld! A creature — a human being — lay beneath the tree. At our approach she rose and gazed wonderingly at us. Had she not done so, I could not have believed her alive. A *very skeleton* emaciated to a terrible degree — yet bloated and swollen in some parts of her body with virulent smallpox. One hand was huge — lumpy and shapeless — and her face! — oh horrible! There was also a wound too, I observed, on her temple, from which oozed the blood. I observed that her bosom was full — as of a nursing woman. My whole soul yearned over her. She gazed at us vacantly — half like an idiot. We all seemed struck motionless at the horrible sight — though still more horrible to relate — some of our men *laughed*! And *my little nurse-maid*! Whom I have just sought for my sweet baby as his nurse. I turned and spoke to her in the bitterness of my soul and indignantly.[40]

Or as one colonial observer would later put it so succinctly, "Native Africans are, as a rule, not cruel, but extraordinarily callous."[41]

Pain was central to how the British came to know their colonial subjects from across the empire and to understand their mission among them. The pain of primitivism (hook swinging, foot binding, genital cutting, tattooing, widow burning) was particularly troubling for its purposeful infliction, as well as its powerful ecstatic and erotic implications.[42] But the pain of illness or of accident in Africa was somehow less upsetting (as it continues to be today), blunted, as it was assumed to be, by the "dulled nerves" of Africans.

Assertions of African insensitivity persisted with support of anecdote, becoming a kind of common sense among many white southern Africans and British visitors.[43] But by the beginning of the twentieth century, such observations were also increasingly lent scientific authority by anthropologists and psychologists. The famous Cambridge Anthropological Expedition to the Torres Straits in 1891 and then the work of R. S. Woodworth at the St. Louis World's Fair in 1904 subjected racialized pain differences to empirical research. This was followed by a series of other such studies. Woodworth explained his methods in the journal *Science* in 1910.

The pain sense is a matter of some interest, because of the fortitude or stolidity displayed by some races towards physical suffering. It may be, and has been conjectured, that the sense for pain is blunt in these races, as it is known to be in some individuals who have allowed themselves to be burned without flinching, and performed other feats of fortitude. The pain sense is tested by applying gradually increasing pressure to some portion of the skin, and requiring the person tested to indicate when he begins to feel pain. Now, as a matter of fact, the results of McDougall on the Papuans, and those of Dr. Bruner and myself on Indians, Filipinos, Africans and Ainu, are in close agreement on this point. Greater pressure on the skin is needed to produce pain in each of these races than in whites.[44]

Racialized differences in pain and other senses were increasingly understood to be an aspect of racial "psychology," reflecting mental traits, a paradigm in which the fact of racialized inferiority in pain sensation was increasingly rendered as scientific fact.[45] Such differences in sensitivity were also hypothesized to arise from fundamental physiological differences. Eighteenth-century Europeans had posited that black skin was tough, thus dulling the pain sense.[46] Such long-standing ideas were repackaged in new language in the 1930s: "It is well known that many African types have strongly developed mesoderm . . . especially connective tissue, and, correlated with this, their sensibility to pain is said to be less."[47]

In 1932, the British social anthropologist C. G. Seligman was still referencing the conclusions of the Torres Expedition and extending such conclusions about racially defined pain sensitivity in his review of the relationship between psychology and anthropology.[48] By the early 1960s, this had fallen out of favor, and the anthropologist Hilda Kuper was finally able to call the assertion that Africans don't feel pain a "stereotype totally unsupported by fact."[49]

As Kuper must have known, psychology began to insert itself more deeply into understandings of pain in the 1950s. Just as neurologists and physiologists concluded that pain perceptions were uniform across races, measured (race-based) reactions to painful stimuli became contested. Controlled settings were weak proxies for the real world of pain, some argued, where subjective anxieties and fears about the meanings of pain helped shape the sensation itself.[50] The conceptual move from pain as purely physiological to pain as a complex experience at once physical, emotional, and social opened the way for culturalist interpretations, like the well-known work of the anthropologist Mark Zoborowski. Zoborowski studied pain in a New York hospital in the 1950s, analyzing differences in the culture of complaint among different American ethnic groups: Jews, Irish, Italians, and so on.[51] Culturalist and psychological analyses of African behavior share a long and entangled history, as many scholars have shown.[52] Where pain is concerned, they merged to call into question African reluctance to perform pain loudly, a phenomenon increasingly understood as a function of culture. In other words, by the late twentieth century, the discussion had shifted from one in which Africans did not feel as acutely, to one in which Africans complained so little. This constellation of ideas in turn often pathologized the patient who dared complain of pain.[53] Pain, as this brief history illustrates, has long been a site of the mutual constitution of race and biomedical practices—a domain where difference was made through social dynamics of expressing, witnessing, and responding to a putatively universal human sensory experience.

In Botswana (formerly Bechuanaland), as Europeans long noted, restraint of expression and maintenance of composure in the face of pain is expected even under the most trying of circumstances.[54] Patients like M and O had therefore developed something of a poetics of endurance. In the oncology ward, at the homes of friends, and in a range of public spaces, indeed throughout my years in Botswana, it often seemed the only person to raise his voice or pound his fist was the German oncologist. This, too, has a history, one of Methodism, no doubt, but also of ritual initiations in which the arts of forbearance were publicly performed, of silent parturients resting between the knees of their mothers-in-law in colonial-era birthing huts, and of hilarious jokes about beating naughty children, among other things.

Historically, Batswana cultivated these forms of forbearance in child rearing and through key sites like initiation camps and birthing huts. Key surgical and obstetrical sites suggest the social quality and significance of pain and its management, as in the oncology ward, where pain was inflicted and experienced with certainty. Until the early to mid-twentieth century, when they were gradually abandoned or reworked, initiation ceremonies were one of the central ritual means by which Batswana perpetuated bodily, intellectual, and social culture simultaneously, transforming unruly youths into disciplined, strong, moral adults. Initiation mirrored birth in complex ways, and the transformative power of pain was harnessed for social reproduction in initiation as it was in childbirth.

In both situations we see a pain drama enacted socially, with bodies physically connected (as they are during procedures in oncology), and certainty about pain accomplished through socialized communication.

A central aspect of *bogwera* (male initiation) was pain-inducing punishment. The young men began their initiation with a formal beating in the *kgotla* (the central village enclosure, where customary court and other meetings were held).[55] Those who had been troublesome youths, who had broken many rules, were on occasion beaten so severely that they died from the wounds. After this preliminary punishment, the initiates were beaten daily in the circumcision camp. Initiates were meant to keep still and silent during all such beatings. The circumcision operation itself was the pinnacle of this practice, as was told to the anthropologist Isaac Schapera.

> Each boy, starting with the chief's son if nobody senior was among them, was led in turn through the lane [of the circumcision camp] by a couple of *bagokane*. As soon as he emerged he was made to stand in front of Rathipana [the circumciser], with his legs outstretched; two *bagokane* held him securely by his arms, "so that he could not stir." The doctor smeared *tshitlo* [made from the burnt ash of the foreskins of the previous regiment, mixed with animal fat] on his forehead, right temple, left temple, and chest; this was done "so that he must no longer think of his home or mother, or be afraid." His loinskin was then removed, also by the doctor. Rathipana . . . immediately took hold of the boy's penis and cut off the foreskin. Meanwhile the men standing around kept shouting or singing loudly "so that the other boys could not hear his cries, but if he cried the men also beat him." . . . The operation was admittedly painful. The older boys, especially, suffered greatly, and it was by no means unusual for one or more of them to die.[56]

Throughout the event, disciplinary pain was imposed on the body and through the body as an integral part of the process, and silence was demanded. Part of the initiate's rebirth as an adult in society meant a demonstrated ability to control his own body on behalf of the commonweal, evidenced by calmly withstanding pain. The initiate's was a profoundly and purposefully socialized body. Yet, as biomedicine and Methodist forms of surgery entered Bechuanaland conjoined, as Paul Landau has argued, pain also began to offer novel possibilities for individuated bodily experience via the knife, a dynamic that might produce laughter.[57]

If initiation was meant to symbolically enact birth, labor itself was also a social drama of pain, forbearance, touching, and witnessing. Surely there were transformations in how women managed births in twentieth-century birthing huts. But the importance of silence, forbearance, and sociality appears to be something of an anchor to the experience.[58] Liv Haram's description of the home-based birth of twins to a thirty-six-year-old woman in the early 1980s is illustrative in this regard.

> The mother-in-law and the *Mmamalome* (father's maternal uncle's wife) are sitting on each side of the laboring woman. The TM (traditional midwife) is sitting right in front of her and they are all facing the woman in labor. Every now and then they comfort her: "*Leka Monyana*" (try, my girl). Another woman answers: "She is trying very hard." Again the TM is advising them to change positions. After some discussion back and forth, they are all in the right position: the mother-in-law is sitting on a chair with her daughter-in-law between her legs supporting her back and holding her arms. The *Mmamalome* is still sitting on the floor beside the woman in labour holding her bent legs. The woman right in front is telling her to push. And she is pushing! Tightening her arms around her mother's legs, she is asking her mother to give her more strength. And the mother does. She clenches her daughter's arms and pushes together with her. They are all pushing. Each of the women twists her face and moves her body as if she herself is giving birth.[59]

Here we see laboring women's pains expressed, read, and responded to in ways that suggest an interactive performance, a collaborative effort. The midwife and other participating women are carefully attuned to nonverbal cues, reading facial expressions to gauge pain. Despite a lack of screaming or moaning, the parturient's pain is not in doubt; it is actively affirmed by everyone in the room, much as Mma H announced O's "botlhoko!" during the bone-marrow biopsy. Pain unfolds as an intersubjective performance of sensation and perception, as patients and caregivers together seek to cool pain into calmness. Yet, as Haram also noted, this poetics of forbearance does not always move intact to hospital delivery rooms, where women labor alone, without female relatives to announce and affirm their pain, and yet where noisy labor might be met with ridicule and chastisement.[60]

PAIN, LAUGHTER, AND SOCIALITY

In the oncology ward, an open ward of twenty beds, there was pain as far as the eye could see, yet it was rarely given voice. But the American doctors and medical students who echoed British missionary complaints of Tswana callousness missed how pain was created as a social fact, and thereby how palliation might proceed. Even pain that remains unvocalized is nonetheless meant to be actively heard, anticipated, and negotiated. The social nature of pain and of embodiment in Botswana places a grave burden on both patient and practitioner. Unlike the individuated patient encased in her envelope of skin, as envisioned through contemporary clinical practice, patients' surgical and other anxieties are as much about maintaining composure in front of others, as about the potentially isolating, individuated experience of bodily pain.

Mma H did her job well by announcing "botlhoko!" so that O did not have to, just as historically women attending to silent parturients announced and enacted the pain of laboring women on their behalf.[61] The entire bone-marrow biopsy is enacted as a drama of few words, but of many meaningful glances, looks, gestures. Bodily contact keeps participants linked in a silent network of social connection, and this socialization is an inherent part of palliation and healing. After his procedure ended, O spoke to me, drawing me into his experience, seeking to socialize his pain. In an inpatient ward, with minimal and highly regulated visiting hours, socializing pain is one of the most significant tasks facing the oncology team, where the ward as a social space must do some of the proxy work of the family.

Botswana's cancer patients usually come to the ward after some months or even years of debilitating pain, fearful for their children, parents, siblings, and lovers as much as for themselves, uncertain of the outcome. They learn of cancer mainly through experience, and a lengthy quest for relief, but they are almost entirely disempowered by rituals of communication and process that seek to shield and protect them from knowledge of their fate. Though they embrace biomedical practice, it is within a context where its hegemony is far from certain. And, of necessity, they bear these procedures with minimal expectation of chemical palliation—a fact that alternately amazes and horrifies us still.

The anxiety of pain in oncology is also the anxiety of death, of orphaning one's children, one's parents, one's siblings, one's lover. In interviews and clinic visits, on questioning, patients and relatives often revealed tremendous depth of concern for the pain of their loved ones. Mothers, aunts, daughters, brothers, fathers, and even entire families might wake in the night to stay with and provide solidarity and comfort to relatives whose pain was intense enough to prevent or interrupt sleep. Young men in their twenties would pause in interviews with me to reflect on how loved and well cared for they were by a favorite aunt or mother who massaged them and sat with them through endless nights of wakeful pain. Patients knew their relatives, motivated by care and love, read them closely, noticing when they became too quiet by day or too restless or mournful at night, seeking out and affirming their pain. In clinic visits where patients failed to mention their own suffering, accompanying relatives would often raise the issue, requesting assistance for their patient.

Callousness toward pain hardly seemed to be the issue when my friend Boitumelo and her sister-in-law Glorious held down Glorious's twenty-three-year-old son and forced morphine down his throat. Bobby, Glorious's son, was dying of a head and neck tumor that had already resulted in the surgical removal of a quarter of his jaw. The tumor was now pushing his eye out of the socket. Profoundly disfigured, perpetually nauseous, and in serious agony, Bobby "just wanted to let the pain kill him," but his mother and aunt felt differently. Unfortunately, by this point in his disease, the maximum dose of oral morphine was only providing him with thirty minutes of relief.

Pain performances, and the existential crises they engender, are subtly gendered. In the rare event that pain was given open voice on the ward, it was usually in the form of cries and tears of women.[62] For young men, by contrast, where silence was required at the limits of human endurance, relentless pain threatened totalizing social rupture. Perhaps it is not surprising that, like Bobby, another young man, P, whose severe Hodgkin's disease was now in partial remission, spoke to me of the suicidal desires that consumed him in the face of his pain. Suicide is a significant problem, particularly among young men in contemporary Botswana, and the issue occupies a prominent role in the contemporary social imaginary.[63] But as P further explained to me, the oncology nurses refused to give up on him. By continually and deeply socializing his pain, they refused him the possibility of enacting relief through self-annihilation. Yet no female patient allowed herself to fantasize about suicide, perhaps given that the price of orphaning her children was simply too high to bear, and perhaps

because of the ways women develop a relationship around pain and social personhood through childbirth.[64] Indeed, many women in oncology
liked to joke about their knowledge of true pain, recalling birth with a
twisted face followed by a knowing laugh.

While patients, like O, usually sat calmly and quietly for bone-marrow
biopsies and aspirates, and even for lung biopsies performed with only
a superficial local anesthetic, when asked directly, they would report
intense burning, or crushing or overwhelming pain. Some writhed or
moaned or wept as the nurses painted gentian violet into open sores in
their anuses or mouths, the sores themselves the product of palliative
radiation treatments. Others sat with teeth clenched as I drove them to
the private hospital across town to get a radiological consult, from which
they carried back to PMH X-rays riddled with the clear white circles of
bone metastases, which explained why they winced each time I hit a
bump in the road. Pain, after all, was what had pushed so many of them
through the health referral system, and into the ward and clinic. But expressions of pain were highly constrained.

There is a complex logic to this that was historically overlooked in
missionary, medical, and anthropological investigations into African
pain. Bodily reserve and continence in the face of pain was a technique
of autopalliation in and of itself. Women learned during labor, and children during the scrapes and accidents of childhood, that becoming overwrought would only intensify pain. In the past, this knowledge was further concretized during the painful tests of ritual initiations. This is a
cultivated disposition, one that is respected as much for its rationality
as for its mark of self-discipline and control. Unfortunately, this logic,
which is never recognized as the product of an intellectual effort to
grapple with the dilemma of pain, produces contradictory effects in contemporary biomedical settings.

PAIN AND LAUGHTER

There was also some absolute hilarity in the face of pain. Patients would
sometimes laugh in interviews when talking about their pain or the pain
of others. Women would reference labor pains and laugh at the image
and the memory. And in the oncology ward and clinic, somewhat to my
surprise, I found (and deeply enjoyed) that laughter was utterly ubiquitous: elderly women who performed outrageous and hysterical pan-

tomimes of the predicament of simultaneous nausea and diarrhea after chemo; middle-aged men who mocked the German mannerisms of the oncologist; young men and women who made deadpan humor out of their hair loss; women with breast cancer who joked about their own fear of death; and then there was the black humor that sometimes followed death, when the oncologist might stride into the ward asking the nurses, "Which of you killed my patient?" Pain, too, was often funny. Laughter in the face of pain may serve to open up a social phenomenology of pain in Botswana's cancer ward.

19 December 2006

A woman patient, who is also a nurse, is lying on the narrow table in the clinic office. She is getting a bone-marrow aspirate, but she doesn't want it. She had it in 2003 and doesn't want it again. "But it takes only two minutes," Dr. P says, insisting. They negotiate as she tries to wheedle out, but he does it quickly, plunging the needle into her sternum, and then she is whimpering—a small wail and it is over as he talks her through, and now everyone is laughing as he explains to me that she is a nurse. The other nurse in the room said, "Sorry, sorry," as the procedure went on. They know each other. "Sorry, my dear." Even the patient laughed at the end when told by her friend that she had cried like a baby. Even ten minutes later another small bout of laughter.

8 January 2007

A young woman, nineteen, with breast lumps. Probably not cancer. She needs an aspirate, and there is much struggle. She keeps wriggling away. Her aunt is laughing so hard at the spectacle, and then says she needs to leave the room. Dr. P asks the aunt to hold her hand. He is doing it very quickly, but the aunt starts laughing and leaves. We all laugh—all of us. She struggles more, and two nursing assistants and the nurse all now are holding her and laughing. It is very comical, and Dr. P is chuckling. Chasing her across the table. "Just a small prick. It is nothing. You must sit still. Why all this fuss? This is not painful, really." Afterward, she finally has it done, lying down and three people helping hold her in place. Dr. P jabs the needle in, pushing it in and out several times to collect any possible calcified material in the lump. She is crying, and the nurse is starting to look a bit annoyed (a young nurse, L, only in her early twenties). And Dr. P asks, "What is wrong? It's over." But she says, "Botlhoko," in a quiet voice and looks injured and angry.

13 March 2007

Dr. P needs to do a fine-needle aspiration on a three-and-a-half-year-old boy. He gives him a banana first, trying to make friends. Then at the nurse's instruction, the boy hands his mother the banana and lies on the table, as Dr. P says, "Small prick," and then jabs the needle into the swollen lymph node on the boy's neck. The kid is screaming and writhing, so the whole thing is chaotic, but the procedure is over in a minute and the nurse, myself, and the nursing assistant have successfully held the boy still enough to get the needle in and out. Afterward, he is crying and screaming and lying on the table demanding his banana: "Ke kopa banana ya me, banana, banana!" His mother gets up and brings it to him. Dr. P is happy that he wants to eat his banana now, feeling certain this will calm him down, and terribly proud that he has thought to give him a piece of fruit. As Dr. P turns his back to empty the syringe onto the slides, the boy comes up behind him and throws the banana at Dr. P's bum with all his might. Everyone collapses to the ground in laughter.

Missionaries, expatriate clinicians, and other observers from the nineteenth century through to the present often took such examples of laughter in the face of the pain of others as a troubling comment on the nature of care and compassion in Botswana, or as a curious cultural artifact.[65] And yet, on closer examination, there appears to be something other than just insensitivity or some exotic culture at play. In fact, the banana-throwing boy became a favorite memory in the clinic, affirming as he did that the procedure *was* painful, though we all (including the patients) were meant to pretend that it wasn't. This laughter was particularly cathartic for the oncologist, who spent his days inflicting pain in the name of care.

Laughter, it seems, has long been a social means for shaping particular forms of autopalliation. Laughter, when it worked, as in the case of the nurse-patient just mentioned, was meant to socialize and redirect patient anxiety into the disposition of calm forbearance that lies at the heart of autopalliation. It was followed by patting or stroking and repetition of "Sorry, sorry," a common way of soothing babies and small children. When laughter didn't work—as in the case of the young woman with the breast aspiration—it served as evidence of the excesses and foolishness of the young, and this, too, was comical. Similarly, women often laughed at and openly mocked the screams and cries of young women in labor,

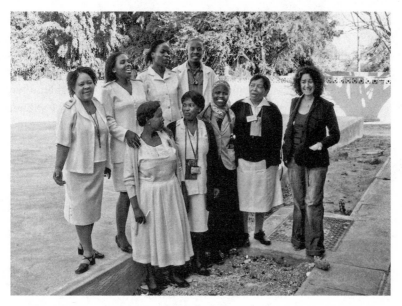

Laughter behind the ward.

the cries signifying that these girls, who thought they were ready for sex, were not yet ready for motherhood.

This is certainly not to suggest that laughter was disingenuous, or an explicit and conscious strategy, but rather to remark on its social effects. If pain, with its potential for isolating embodiment, threatens social rupture, laughter offers the prospect of reestablishing embodied sociality. I don't intend to be overly functionalist here. Laughter is often a spontaneous response to an overwhelming experience, not a response that emerges out of diligence and forethought. And laughter can be sadistic, it can be thin and false, it can be an expression of nervousness and discomfort. Laughter, like all emotional experiences and expressions, has a cultural logic, and one can decode this logic, though at the risk of taking all the fun out of the laughter itself. Some of its joy, no doubt, derives from its irreverence—laughter in the oncology ward often served to acknowledge the utter absurdity of misfortune. This is not unique to Botswana, and while I was there, I was often reminded not only of Bakhtin, but also of keeping my friend Matthew company while he sat on the chemo drip for the liver cancer that killed him in 1994 at age twenty-eight. When the nurse would check in and ask if he was OK, he would reply, "Nothing to worry about here, just a little cancer," and somehow it was absolutely hilarious to us.[66] But laughter is also a form of social expression, and tracing its effects around pain reminds us that pain, too, is social. It distributes responsibilities, including to the pained subject. Laughter often comes in moments when cultural norms fail to be enacted—the patient fails to keep silent, the doctor fails to maintain his authority—and thus, in its recognition of the absurd, laughter reinforces the norm, by socializing it. In none of these scenarios does anyone laugh alone.

Of course laughter can be cruel, as when R, a long-standing ᴋs patient, cried all the way back to her bed from the toilet, where her defecation had been painful. Her overwrought cries, so out of place on the ward, were met with cynical laughter by the nurses. But R had a long history in oncology, and though she could be wickedly funny in her own right, often cracking jokes that had us howling with laughter, she was also "naughty," as one fellow patient put it, drinking to excess, sleeping with many men, and even joking about making a sexual advance on her own brother. "She likes this hospital too much,"* a nursing assistant commented, meaning that R was not taking enough responsibility for her own well-being. Pain and laughter, as fundamental and at times overwhelming bodily experiences, point to the potential for both positive social connection *and* profoundly isolating social alienation, and they often bundle together or cascade out from one another for just this reason. They can counteract and balance or accelerate one another; in tandem they reveal something of the strength of social embodiment.

In Tswana medicine and popular thought, pathological experience is at least in one key sense the outcome of social rupture and antagonism. Thus, pain in this configuration is already a fundamentally social phenomenon, and palliation, like healing, attempts to resocialize, in this case through the benign intimacy of companionship, physical touch, and, of course, laughter. This socialization and intimacy that laughter provides is especially critical in the face of cancer. In Botswana, where cancer is still a somewhat novel experience that people are just now trying to make sense of, some (perhaps many) people understand cancer to be a potentially communicable disease, so that patient utensils, bedding, and space are often kept separate. Because of the constraints of the health system, many cancer patients in pain are also suffering from disfiguring tumors or amputations, overflowing saliva (among those whose throats are entirely blocked by esophageal tumors), and the necrotic stench of tumors that have broken through the skin and exposed rotting flesh. Sociality is potentially tenuous for these patients, and laughter all the more powerful for its potential not only to facilitate autopalliation, but also to strengthen and animate benign social connectivity, which *is* healing and care for Batswana.

Laughter, of course, is not the only form of popular response to pain in this culture of silent expression. Nor did callousness seem to be at issue when S, a woman with stage 4 metastatic breast cancer, began crying out in pain in the ward. In my field notes I wrote:

> *After lunch in the ward, S—the woman with metastatic breast cancer who got chemo in a lumbar puncture on Friday—is really crying out in pain. This is such an unusual sound in the onco ward. Drs. A and P and Mma M all hurry over. She has a crushing pain in the head and wants to vomit. Dr. A doubles her dose of pethidine and then there is a question: does she have meningitis? She will get antibiotics just in case, etc. But there is a deep and swift reaction to her crying out in pain. I am impressed.*

Though pain threatens to isolate an individual in his or her body, ideally (if not always in practice) every effort is made to socialize it, through active affirmation of its presence, through palliation, through laughter, through bodily contact.

Over time it became clear that the oncology ward was a particularly rich social world, one whose logic escaped expatriate and Batswana observers who complained of the callousness of Batswana nursing staff. To be sure, there were some patients who were ignored or generally lost in the shuffle of clinical activity, and others who were perceived as irritating in some way, which may have affected their care. But sweeping indictments of a Batswana culture of compassion don't quite fit this very complex social space. Some nurses were cancer patients themselves, I learned, and others had watched their own parents die in the very ward where they now worked. Among the general flow of work, nurses actively cared for cousins, nieces, neighbors, friends, patients who began as strangers but became incredibly dear, and, of course, patients they learned to loathe.

Many patients, when I asked them if pain had a purpose, remarked on its ability to enhance their empathetic and perceptive capacities. They replied that it had given them new insight into their fellow citizens in the "country of the sick," as Susan Sontag would have put it. Their empathetic and perceptive abilities deepened, some patients remarked that the purpose of pain was to cause them to remember God and to recognize and care for others in times of suffering. Again, this mirrors the logics of bongaka and Christian healing prophecy, in which many healers are called to their task through crises of personal suffering that enable them to recognize empathetic and perceptive abilities that they can then develop through study.[67] For many veteran patients, the experience of traumatic pain opens them to perceiving it in others without a need for language. Doubt was not at issue. Instead, some felt that they had to turn away when they now witnessed the pain of others—it was simply too exquisite, too intense a mnemonic for their own agony, now that they had such a clearly embodied sense of what a grimace, a cringe, a tightly held brow indexed. Some found themselves comparing their pain to that of others they met in the ward or while waiting in the clinic or elsewhere, measuring their own pain against the presumed suffering of others, "placing it on the scale to weigh." In this way they either consoled themselves, openly acknowledging the pain of a fellow patient, or affirmed their sense that their own suffering was indeed extreme.

In conversations with Tswana healers, I found that it was nearly impossible to talk about pain as pain, to imbue it with ontological import, much less to historicize it. Pain, it seemed, could not be separated from cause. It continually collapsed back into its underlying pathology, even when I tried steering the conversation toward the pain of flogging or of stubbing one's toe, experiences that I assumed were not pathological.[68] Tswana healers had clearly absorbed and reworked various biomedical concepts, entities, technologies, and schemes, talking to me about blood, germs, brains, and other organs in ways that were sometimes substantially different from similar conversations I had had with healers a decade earlier. A few had been through HIV training meetings set up for African healers by biomedically oriented primary hospitals and NGOs, but none of this facilitated a dialogue about pain. Surely this fact, this total situatedness of pain, its refusal to be separated from the flow of pathological experience is in itself meaningful, reinforcing the sense that I have tried to convey of the already complex and compound social, bodily, and emotional sensibility around pain that is manifest in the ward.

PROVISIONAL CONCLUSIONS

I have tried to suggest in this chapter that pain is a fundamental social experience in Botswana's cancer ward and in the hospital more broadly, one that both drives patients into the institution and is created by the practices of the institution itself. Yet, despite the fact that pain is one of the central animating forces of biomedical care in Africa, of which Botswana's cancer ward is but one instantiation, the biomedical technologies and techniques of palliation are sparse and put to uneven and uncertain use.

Pain reveals the intensely social nature of the ward. Through pain, patients know that something critical is happening to them, and thus they must find ways to express this experience to their caregivers. But the mechanisms and semantics of acceptable expression are particular and often difficult to achieve. Into the breach of expression comes laughter, a social experience for reinstantiating and reestablishing community in moments of terrible anxiety and duress.

CODA ON A FAILED LEARNING CURVE

30 January 2007

In the opposite bed from Michael in men's surgical lay M, the man with the botched amputation, which is now scheduled to be cleaned up and bone removed, etc. He is still here. M saw Dr. P and beckoned him. Then, after Dr. P left, he grabbed the male nurse who was with me and asked him for pain meds. "The pain is too much—I need an injection." The nurse says he can't have an overdose of pethidine. But he also hasn't looked at the file. I am not sure if he knows when the last dose was. The patient says, "Maybe I can take it at noon," and the nurse agrees. I am not sure why he is still on pethidine and not on morphine. The nurse doesn't seem concerned about this. He wants to ask me instead about job opportunities in the United States. M, empowered by my presence [in this context, where my whiteness causes the nurse to mistake me for an American doctor], is learning to ask for relief. Yet the effort comes up short.

SIX

After ARVs, During
Cancer, Before Death

Batswana are learning rapidly about the power of certain biomedical technologies such as chemotherapy or radiotherapy in easing suffering and potentially staving off death. Yet these same goods are proving more complicated, less miraculous than is hoped. Cancer deaths expose the ironies and problems lying at the intersection of technoscientific and international development progress narratives, whereby citizens of Botswana, Batswana, having seized hold of their futures through ARVs, now long for a political economy in which they can inherit the power of clinical oncology. There is urgent need for well-funded and well-run *public* oncology settings across Africa. However, while political and economic hopes for improved care are crucial, developmental fantasies that hinge on improved technological access, whether in the form of ARVs or chemotherapy, will not allow Batswana to avoid the contradictions and dilemmas that accompany high-tech medicine. While there have been critical advances over the past several decades, the therapeutic space where better detection and treatment make a difference in terms of patient futures is nonetheless smaller than we might hope.[1] So in one sense, Botswana is a more "utopian" setting for oncology, in that the simple provision of clinical services is in itself a form of rapid progress, and yet the ambiguities of this progress are rapidly felt.[2]

Novel technologies burst onto complicated political and economic landscapes, generating new desires and hopes. But as these technologies become normative and embedded in complex and often dysfunctional infrastructural fields, their ambiguities are revealed, and the challenges of practice become more burdensome, spawning both political critique and individual creativity.[3] Perhaps nowhere is this ambiguity more apparent than in death.[4]

In the oncology ward of PMH fundamental clinical ethics are at play in the troubled and deeply equivocal moral grounds on which doctors, nurses, family members, and patients attempt to sustain commitments to each other's well-being even as they occupy different positions of power. Yet in Botswana, a country with universal access to healthcare for citizens, and with a historically deep and explicit understanding of care as a densely social dynamic, we encounter a particular pragmatics and an ethos of clinical medicine that at least partially diverges from what the philosopher Annemarie Mol calls "the choice model" of healthcare.[5] In the PMH oncology ward, patients are always already members of collectivities, distributive justice (or the ethics of rationing) takes on *the* overshadowing urgency, and decision making for the end-stage terminally ill is socially distributed rather than premised on notions of individual patient autonomy.

THE PROBLEM OF BEDS

Entering PMH, one immediately is struck by the degree to which demand for care is outstripping capacity. This is a relatively well-funded hospital, compared to many African institutions, and it sits atop a broader set of well-distributed primary and provincial hospitals, and an extensive network of clinics. But, as we have seen in relation to the nursing crisis, it is also a place where a profound AIDS epidemic and three decades of population growth have taken their toll on an already overstretched public hospital. Plans for construction of a more up-to-date and capacious institution are now under way, as part of the establishment of the country's first medical school. But for the foreseeable future, PMH remains Botswana's hospital of resort.

Anyone lucky enough to be arriving at PMH by car, as I often was, will encounter the problem of space almost immediately. The hospital parking lot is perpetually full during business hours, with cars parked in the middle of the lanes, blocking those already in the designated spaces, perched on the curbs and cement embankments, and with drivers gunning between parking lanes in reverse at the first sign that someone might be vacating a spot. I often caught a ride with a Motswana surgical officer who lived near me. Fearing the wrath of the Ukrainian thoracic surgeon, his superior, he would circle the parking lot in an act of desperate futility, before ramming his silver 1998 Toyota Tazz atop, say, a small embankment next to one of the corrugated tin tuck shops that line the parking lot selling snacks, toilet paper, and cool drinks, and then fleeing toward the surgical ward in an effort to arrive before the start of morning meeting. Dr. P, I might note, had a habit of driving his own Tazz at relatively high speed through the back gate of the hospital (an entrance reserved for deliveries), past the morgue, over the dirt yard between the minor theater and the wall that separated it from the street, and parking it on the dirt, essentially in the middle of hospital grounds, near the back door of oncology.

Entering the hospital from the proper parking lot, one passes the surgical, gynecological, and medical clinics, with their vast communal waiting room packed with patients. In the morning the queue to register snakes far down the breezeway toward the Accident and Emergency Department. In 2004, this 507-bed hospital had an average admission rate of 650 patients, and there were days where it was operating at 200 percent capacity. Since then things have eased slightly—but only slightly. In the surgical, medical, and obstetrics and gynecology wards, all beds are perpetually full, with narrow gurneys packed along the hallways. Former storage closets and duty rooms have been converted to accommodate patients, and many patients must lie on the floor. The one exception is the "private ward" with its semiprivate rooms, for which patients pay a fee (about $10) for each night in residence. This is the ward that Dr. P calls "Marx's revenge," because this sliver of private space often proves dangerous. There are no call buttons, and visiting hours are brief. With patients hidden in private rooms rather than being visible in an open ward, emergencies sometimes go unnoticed until it is too late.

The premium on bed-space in the cancer ward has tremendous implications for how and where Botswana's cancer patients will die. The ward, like the rest of the hospital, is perpetually full, often with extra beds or gurneys packed in where possible. The pressure on space structures care. Many ambulatory patients on chemotherapy are given push injections, since there is little room for outpatients to sit on drips, much less to accommodate the lounge chairs of American chemo centers. Batswana women with breast cancer who have just received doxorubicin and cyclophosphamide must make their way to the central station and pack onto buses for their journeys home, dizzy and vomiting into their headscarves or into a precious, bright red, plastic biohazard bag sneaked to them by a nurse or a visiting ethnographer. But some chemotherapy regimens require pre- and post-hydration with intravenous fluids and include drugs that need to run in intravenously over many hours, frequently taking three to five days for completion of the treatment course. Patients on these regimens need beds in order to receive treatment. Delays are dangerous. And many of the PMH oncology patients have risen before dawn in homes as far away as the western rim of the Kalahari to journey several hours to join the queue in oncology. They cannot be sent back without treatment. Many would not find funds or clinic-based transport for a return journey the next day, and such journeys are arduous for the sick. Cancer illnesses and treatments produce side-effects that often require unexpected hospitalizations, and when such patients arrive, they must be accommodated.

Likewise, the only radiotherapy unit in the country is located in the Gaborone Private Hospital, across town from PMH. The government pays for public patients to receive radiation treatments at GPH. In addition, the Cancer Association of Botswana (a small NGO) maintains a small, twenty-bed, "interim home" dormitory in the city for ambulatory patients who live too far away to commute for daily radiation. Yet the interim home is perpetually full, so overflow patients and those receiving radiation who are not ambulatory or who are weak enough to require more extensive nursing services often occupy beds in PMH oncology. Bottlenecks at the radiotherapy machine, which are frequent, produce bottlenecks in bed-space at PMH oncology.

The numbers of cancer patients in the country continue to rise, and in June of 2008, when I returned to PMH after a year away, Dr. P, the oncologist, was still actively staving off the prospect of housing patients on the already crowded floor, despite tremendous problems at the radiotherapy unit, where staff had quit in anger over their conditions of employment. Supported by his outreach efforts, peripheral hospitals had begun providing basic chemotherapy for patients with Kaposi's sarcoma, the most commonly diagnosed cancer, thus easing up clinic and ward space. Yet even this could not stem the tide of patients. Cancer patients were now occupying an entire five-bed cubicle in the perpetually under-occupied Eye Ward at PMH (the *only* under-occupied ward), and others originally admitted to the surgical, medical, orthopedic, and gynecological wards began and often completed their chemotherapy treatments there, while awaiting transfer to oncology. In other words, oncology was slowly spilling out of the ward and competing for space throughout an already profoundly overcrowded hospital.

TRIAGE OF THE TERMINALLY ILL

The shortage of beds means that, ideally, those who are dying — those for whom Dr. P has determined that active oncology treatment has little left to offer — are sent home during the window of time when they are ambulatory.[6] It means patients are sometimes loaded onto ambulances, some of which are no more than glorified pick-up trucks, to bring them to a primary hospital several hours' drive away, with their final IV bag of post-chemo hydration still hanging, even if they and their relatives and the clinical staff would prefer for them to remain at PMH. And it means that some patients are given abbreviated courses of outpatient chemo with a push injection, rather than the standard in-patient IV course if there is no bed available. It also leads to social tensions, miscommunications, and often crises, as relatives, nurses, and doctors do not always understand or accept Dr. P's sometimes opaque triage logic, much less agree on who is dying and who is not, and how imminent or certain those deaths are.

In the midst of such debates Dr. P often said he could not give a bed based on social problems. He allocated beds based on treatment logics. Yet the biological and the social were not so easily peeled apart, and ultimately even the biological was open to reinterpretation given the instability of the technological field. Mma M, by contrast, realized that the patients with the fewest committed relatives to care for them at home were also those who lacked relatives to advocate for their continued admission in the ward, a terribly irony. "This is why we are always arguing on behalf of the patients without relatives to care for them. They get discharged but not [those with aggressive families advocating for them]. It is we nurses who will speak on their behalf," she explains.

And this is all happening in a place which is intimate enough that actual lives are being weighed against one another. No one has the luxury here of abstract ethical reasoning. One Friday in March of 2007 the nurses were simmering with anger when they realized that Mary would have to be sent home. They wanted Fatty, a wealthy woman with bone cancer and demanding relatives, to go instead. But Dr. P insisted otherwise. Mary was so sweet, and we all knew her last few months would be gruesome. She had a massive, terminal cancer of the vulva, which had eaten away much flesh and left her stinking and barely able to walk. There was no way she and her sister could care properly for the wound in their tiny shack in the nearby urban slum, and stinking as she did, Mary would have few visitors to help. But it would clearly take her several months to die, and Dr. P stood his ground. "No, Mary must go. We cannot give a bed or she will become unable to move and we will lose that bed for months." And so off she went that afternoon, trundling down the corridor with wide-set legs, wincing in pain, but politely making her good-byes.

In other words, it means that when Beauty, the forty-nine-year-old woman with end-stage laryngeal cancer, whose throat was swollen shut from radiotherapy, arrived, deeply dehydrated and in extreme misery, with her anguished husband, she could not be admitted to oncology, despite her husband's understandable, but quiet anger and frustration. Instead, they were forced to find friends with a car to immediately transport her to the primary hospital in her home village, some four hours' drive away, after a brief rehydration intervention in the chemo room. Being shunted away was an assertion that active treatment was now futile and that Beauty would certainly die soon. Dr. P had prepared her husband for this over a series of conversations in the four preceding months. But this did not soften the moment itself. Dr. P was giving up on Beauty. Her husband was not yet prepared to do the same. Hours after they left, Dr. P was still upset, certain she was dying, but uncertain he had done the right thing in sending Beauty away. Then again, as he repeatedly told himself (and me), he had no other choice. He simply couldn't give her a bed.

There are, of course, many patients who do die in the ward. Some arrive in reasonable shape, but then develop complications and become too sick to move. Others arrive in dire condition and die in the ward before the next scheduled date for an ambulance returning to their home area. Many, like Mary, are from Gaborone, and therefore cannot be referred to a primary hospital. But nonetheless every effort is made to deflect dying patients back to their homes or to peripheral hospitals within the system. This logic suggests that beds are reserved for those who require a *doctor's* care, particularly for those whose lives might be extended by chemotherapeutic or radiation treatment. Yet in practice many patients require hospitalization because of their need for professional, intensive *nursing* care, especially given the prevalence of necrotic wounds, and the intense pain and discomfort of a cancer death. Knowing this, nurses sometimes oppose Dr. P in fraught discussions about whom to discharge. In the ward the zero-sum game of bed-space means decisions are anything but abstract.

Nursing cancer patients at home without clinical support is extremely challenging. There is a history to the new urgency and efforts by which some relatives try to achieve a hospital-based death for their patient. In this, the second decade of the AIDS epidemic, who in Botswana has not lived in a home where a relative or two or three lay dying? No one is naïve about death and what it looks, feels, sounds, and smells like. There are some people, to be sure, who are exhausted by this and want to shift the responsibility of care for the dying onto the state via the hospital. But there are also many others with deep regrets or haunting questions not only about the facts or causes of death, but perhaps much more about the stark agony in which their relatives died. Could they have done more? Could the hospital have offered something if they had been able to push their patient into PMH or raised funds for a private doctor? These memories animate ongoing attempts by relatives to achieve admission.[7]

Those from outside the city no longer on active treatment are discharged for follow-up by their local primary hospital or clinic. Yet with morphine and codeine—the two strong analgesics for outpatients on the country's essential drug list—concentrated at PMH, such sites prove poor substitutes for the oncology ward itself in managing end-of-life care. This happened to Mma Pula, a woman I visited who was dying of cervical cancer in her home. Mma Pula was living with a massive post-radiation fistula, such that urine, feces, and blood were all coming out of her vagina. She was in severe pain and had an intense fear of eating, since defecation was so agonizing. Her clinic card showed she was on ibuprofen. Morphine had been ordered at PMH, but it is not stocked at the primary hospitals, so her only hope for meaningful pain relief was to find a way back into PMH for help. A poor woman heading a household of ten, who had fallen through the cracks in the health system, her fantasies about money were fantasies about PMH and pain relief. She told me, "If I were someone who would be rich or whatever, each time that I would go to the hospital I would go straight to PMH, because they are the ones who are actually doing something [about the pain]."*

UNCERTAIN FUTURES

Amid the relative scarcity of tertiary care, and the tremendous pain and angst of a cancer illness, it is not surprising that many patients and their relatives seek to secure a future through more therapies, more hospital time, more admissions. For them, progress after ARVs is about pursuing more high-tech medicine. Yet in Botswana, where the majority of patients are diagnosed with already advanced disease and where their treatment might be further complicated by an HIV co-infection, prognosis is often poor. One of the difficulties facing the oncologist is the knowledge that even if there were more beds, drugs, expertise, and machines, many of the patients in the PMH cancer ward would still be terminally ill. Dr. P must help the growing population of patients and relatives maintain hope in oncology as a technomedical pursuit that can extend life and ease suffering. But he must also regularly acknowledge individual instances of therapeutic futility, especially since this acknowledgment is critical to the rationing of care. In PMH oncology this is accomplished through a culture of medical paternalism that operates in two registers. First, the oncologist is recognized to wield powerful expertise and knowledge that exceeds the understanding of laypersons, and he is expected to do so in the benign service of vulnerable patients. Second, he is charged with the ethical rationing of beds, goods, and services. Relatives (more so than terminally ill patients themselves) provide one check on both dimensions of the oncologist's power through their urgent requests for care.

In Botswana's cancer ward, as in many other parts of PMH, future-making through technomedicine melds paternalism and self-determination into a fragile if necessary combination. Patients must place their trust in the oncologist and his therapies, even when the nature of the problem and its outcome are far from certain. They must be disciplined, yet agentive and self-determined through the rigors of therapy. That is, until the oncologist determines that they have entered the terminal phase of illness. From that moment forward, much of their autonomy will be stripped and socially distributed to their kin through customs of prognostication that allow for frank, if brief, discussions with relatives, but not with patients.

In 2007 Mothusi, a really marvelous young man with end-stage cancer, lay shivering and sweating, the feeding tube exposed on his bare abdomen. He cringed in pain as Dr. A, the Egyptian medical officer, pushed the four tubes of chemotherapeutic drugs into the central intravenous line implanted in his chest. He lay back exhausted and shaking, and prepared for the onslaught of nausea and fatigue that would soon follow. Mothusi had arrived in the ward by ambulance on a hot, crowded day from South Africa, where he had been hospitalized while attending university. The doctors there had sent him home to Botswana, as a terminal case. Fortunately, his parents raised the funds for him to be housed in the private ward of PMH and so bed-space was not at issue. The tumor was so large it blocked his throat entirely, so that he could not even swallow his own saliva. He was anxious that he might be given a tracheostomy—something he very much did not want.

In the counseling session immediately after his arrival, Mothusi's parents were surprised to learn from Dr. P that the doctors in South Africa were certain the case was terminal. The South Africans had failed to explain the situation to them, a not uncommon turn of events in which private doctors failed to deliver pessimistic prognostic information, leaving this for the public clinician. Mothusi's parents wanted everything possible done for their son—couldn't Dr. P at least "give chemo" or "scan him"? "We know, doctor, that you will try your best."* Because of the incomplete medical records from South Africa, there was at least a small chance that Mothusi, despite the advanced stage of his disease might respond to treatment. So Dr. P acceded to his parents' insistence that he receive an aggressive course of chemotherapy, that the oncology team not give up on him. Then over the next several weeks, in various counseling sessions, he began to lay out where the road would end. Before long, I found myself, like his mother, somehow certain that Mothusi would be different, engaging in what Joan Didion calls "magical thinking."[8] He was just too wonderful to die. I am embarrassed to write that on more than one occasion I put an impossible pressure on Dr. P, insisting that he simply would have to save Mothusi, that he *must* cure him completely. Dr. P trod a careful path between hope and honesty with me. But I had begun to believe my own faith.

Chemo was quite a miserable experience, but it did at least initially provide Mothusi with some relief, even as he suffered its side-effects. Dr. P, Dr. A, and I all knew there was little chance that the chemo would significantly extend Mothusi's life, but it was impossible not to hope along with his parents. And so with the CT scanner broken, we clung to and debated the ambiguities of his X-rays—were the metastases in his lungs shrinking, or was the exposure of the film different? Yet life on chemotherapy was at times agonizing. For three solid days after the painful injections, Mothusi would face totalizing nausea, dizziness, and intense exhaustion. Then, five or six days later, when his white cell count would plummet, he would succumb to a series of nasty infections in his chest, intestinal tract, and ears. Some days he lay sweating with tumor fever. He had received heavy doses of radiation while he was abroad, and the chemo produced a "recall effect," thus intensifying his symptoms.

This is not to say that he found no pleasure in life. He listened to music. Countless friends and relatives came to visit him. He read the newspapers. His mother and father were there every day, and some weekends he was even allowed to go home on a hospital furlough. He joked with his doctors, his nurses, and the ethnographer who followed them around. For his parents, Mothusi embodied the emergence of an aspirational ethos of patient care in Botswana, where "First World," high-tech medicine hovers as an imagined promise against which Batswana evaluate risks and imbue value in the lives of patients. It was also their decision not to inform him of his prognosis, though I am quite sure he knew there was little hope. Then, several weeks after he arrived at PMH, Mothusi choked to death in the middle of the night, as Dr. P, called in from home, watched the surgical officer give him the emergency tracheotomy he had feared. Did it matter that he died with a scalpel jutting out of his throat? Did it matter that his mother would survive him knowing that she hadn't given him up without a fight? Was this a charade of therapeutic futility? Or a necessary exercise in hope? Would his mother have charted a different course if high-tech medicine were not so novel? Would Mothusi himself if he'd been the one to choose? Did care fail here? Did clinical ethics?

As death grows certain, patients like Mothusi develop tacit knowledge of their prognoses. These are not sudden deaths, they are agonizing processes—and the phenomenology of dying is larded with its own insights. Patients might tell a nurse or the visiting ethnographer that they are afraid for their futures, afraid they might die, even as they hope she might contradict them. But rarely did anyone say such things to Dr. P. He would tell them he was buying time, that he could treat but not cure their problems. But he never said, "You are dying," and they never asked. Occasionally those who were not yet dying expressed a fear of death to

Dr. P. This would become a great joke between patient and doctor. "Ah! You! Here comes my patient who thought I would just let him die! Are you dead?" "No, not yet!" And everyone would laugh heartily at the absurdity of such a fear.

The lack of death talk among the terminally ill didn't mean that patients were not preoccupied with their prognoses. Of course they were. My interviews often turned into counseling sessions, and nurses often spent time managing the anxieties of patients about their futures, and those of their children. Death was always present—but words were about trying, and I learned to use the myopic grammar of dying on the ward. As patients questioned me about their futures, I replied in the present continuous, truncating time's horizon.

As they enter the end stage, patients often begin to develop tacit knowledge of their prognoses. This might be based on their own assessments of their physical declines, social clues (like extra efforts made to arrange hospital visits by school-age children, by previously estranged relatives, or those who live far away and must raise travel fare), and, for those who have figured out the basic contours of oncology over time, the realization that no more chemo, radiation, or surgery will be forthcoming. When patients were frank with Dr. P, and asked pointed questions, Dr. P was truthful with them, though he strongly resisted giving clear temporal frameworks in such prognostic conversations. But rarely do patients initiate or participate in open discussion with the oncologist about the terminal nature of their illnesses and the futility or benefit of various therapeutic options.[9] It was rare for patients to present Dr. P with direct questions about death or temporal horizons.

Usually, Dr. P. would summon relatives into his office alone, to discuss the patient still lying in the ward. Or during a clinic visit, he would instruct the patient to remain waiting in his office, while he took the accompanying relatives, the clinic nurse, and me into the treatment room for a quick prognostic conversation. In such meetings, termed "counseling sessions," Dr. P was direct. "The situation is a disaster," he would say in his characteristic German accent. Or "It is absolutely hopeless." Or "Yes, he is better now, but it won't last. It will not last." As Dr. P explained when I questioned him, it is not that he tells the patient nothing of the prognosis. "I do, I tell them we are buying time, or that something cannot be cured, only treated. But when the situation is totally hopeless, then I do not. There are no rules—but the one rule I follow is that I *always* talk frankly to the relatives. I always tell them the entire truth."* Patients, for their part, took their own meanings from their absence at such meetings.

Dr. P, like many oncologists in Africa, felt it was important to be blunt with relatives, so that they did not expend precious resources taking their patient to private clinicians in a futile hope of finding a cure for their loved one.[10] Yet, despite Dr. P's directness in these conversations, relatives sometimes pushed back against his terminal prognosis and triage logic. In this context, where experience with the short-term power of oncology in shrinking painful tumors combines with widespread experience with ARVs, terminal prognoses can seem less certain. And so requests for more intervention, more therapy, more care were often part of such discussions, requests that Dr. P then weighed in relationship to the specifics of the case and the availability of resources. So, too, the repeated refrain among relatives and patients alike, "We know, doctor, that you are trying your best," served as a continual reminder of the ethics at play. Patients and relatives might not have expected to make therapeutic choices, but they did require demonstrated energy and commitment from their oncologist.

Dr. P was not alone in sharing terminal prognoses with relatives rather than with patients. Until recently, this was the norm in most of the world, and it continues today, even though an emphasis on patient autonomy has been emerging in some countries since the 1970s, reorienting the logic of the clinical encounter.[11] Over the course of our time together, I often debated with Dr. P the ethics of his form of prognostication. As someone steeped in a contemporary American ethos of patient autonomy, I was deeply troubled by the lack of direct communication with the patient herself. In particular I was distressed by the times when Dr. P would urge relatives not to tell the patient what had been discussed, rather than let them draw their own conclusions based on their knowledge of the patient. These norms, I pointed out, risk perpetuating a southern African history of colonial medicine that was highly paternalistic, facilitating potentially harmful and exploitative practices. On several occasions I accused Dr. P of a crude paternalism. This was a criticism he was willing to take. Yet, as I came to see, even if I could not bring myself to agree, his approach, developed over the many years he spent working in Zimbabwe before coming to Botswana, was the product of serious effort to weigh the exigencies of the situation at hand and to chart what he saw as the most efficacious course. Was this paternalism in the sense that it denied information? Or was that kind of paternalism necessary for *care* by someone in the lonely and unenviable position of envisioning possible futures of the patients in ways that they could not, given the novelty of cancer in Botswana and the post-ARV sense of therapeutic possibility held by some relatives? If it was paternalism in that second sense, then it was a paternalism wielded on the one hand to push some patients into life-saving treatment that they initially resisted and later celebrated. And it was a paternalism inherent to the rationing of clinical time, resources, and bed-space, which already competed with autonomy in troubling ways.

Paternalism, if we are to call it that, lies somewhere at the heart of international (now global) health—and it can be very dangerous. From the perils of medical experimentation to outright coercion, at its worst medical paternalism threatens to foreclose the types of lay questioning, critique, and self-determination that are necessary to check the tremendous power clinicians and policy-makers have over the sick. In recent decades, increased patient autonomy has been posited as progress, by those seeking rights as patients and by ethicists alike, as the proper response to the potential problems posed by medical paternalism. Yet, in Botswana, a surging interest in technomedicine as progress has not been accompanied by an easy turn to autonomy.

Certainly, there is a right to health, and activists throughout the developing world have worked hard to try to secure and enact those rights in a meaningful way. But global health is also, and perhaps predominantly, driven by a feeling among experts that they know which afflictions matter and how to handle them, to the extent that they sometimes cajole or counsel or frighten or entice or force people into conforming to biomedical therapies and behavioral models.[12] One man I interviewed hadn't realized that the surgeons in South Africa were going to remove his larynx and give him a tracheostomy, until he awoke in a ward and felt his neck. Such stories are not uncommon in this part of the world, where until recently African patients, including many Batswana, received their care in hospitals located in institutionally racist states (South Africa, Southern Rhodesia, South West Africa). There is an ugly history in southern Africa, of which all Batswana are well aware. However, at least in this oncology ward, this ugly history is not the whole story.

Meanwhile, Tswana notions of personhood and the ethos of care and responsibility, all of which are socially distributed, are manifest in this logic of tacit knowledge for the subject and explicit knowledge for the relatives. Time and again, Batswana affirmed to me their commitment to the social displacement of terminal prognostication onto relatives. Many were appalled that doctors in the United States (or the United Kingdom or Australia) tell patients that they are dying. The anthropologist Fred Klaits has described with great nuance the importance of speech acts in Botswana, explaining how words and sentiments are understood to have powerful effects on others and thus must be deployed with care in ways that build up positive sentiments between people, a lesson we Americans might profitably attend.[13] And many people with whom I spoke felt that direct language about death in a clinical encounter could cause patients to "give up" and die earlier than necessary. Words can kill. Indeed, in Botswana, to tell someone that they would die was the antithesis of care and resonated with forms of social pathos like witchcraft. If properly chosen, of course, words can also comfort; they are fundamental to care.[14] I also think acceptance of the social distribution of prognoses was an ethical stance taken by patients, a refusal to be isolated from a broader social collectivity charged with their care. It was also an ethical stance taken by relatives, who wiped away tears as they prepared themselves to shoulder the burden of discretion for the sake of their patient.

Culture, of course, is never monolithic. A handful of young Batswana doctors and some university students with whom I spoke were troubled by these rituals of future-making. It is quite likely that the widespread stress on patient confidentiality in the AIDS industry (even as that confidentiality is regularly breached, and even as public disclosure of HIV status is encouraged), that the public interest in rights and emphasis on self-determination at the national level, and that shifting social norms of care-giving and reliance are beginning to produce changes in normative values around rituals of prognostication. When Naniso was dying of non-Hodgkin's lymphoma in the private ward, she acknowledged and openly discussed her death, requesting that a social worker be sent to her room to help her manage her feelings of depression and loss. Her roommate, Linda, on the other hand, whose intestinal tract was entirely obstructed by metastatic disease from the recurrence of her ovarian cancer, deflected any discussion of how the treatment was failing. She told Dr. P repeatedly, as he implied the futility of further treatment, that she knew he was trying his best and that she was in God's hands. She died ten days after her friend.

What the debates in the United States around patient autonomy often skate over is the very real investment that relatives as daily caregivers and as loved ones have in treatment decisions. Paternalism, in the colonial sense of coercion, is no less problematic in PMH than it was in hospitals in the United States, where it was openly challenged by rights-based movements in the 1970s. It might even be more so in this African hospital named for a European princess. But any medical system is built on the premise that patients cannot fully care for themselves. Therefore, paternalism in the sense of moral obligation inherent to the acknowledged, structural inequality between caregivers and care-receivers is necessary in order to provide care for those who are vulnerable. This extends to those who provide care in the home (relatives) as well as those who provide care in institutions (doctors and nurses).

We cannot romanticize the social, even as we grapple with its primacy. Social relations are complicated. In Setswana, relatives who arrive at the home of a patient are counseled as to the diagnosis and condition of the afflicted. Relatives arrive at the hospital expecting these same forms of disclosure to hold. Yet control over illness narratives can become a key arena of social contestation within families.[15] As Dr. S, a Motswana medical officer, commented to me, recognizing that not all relatives were equally well situated or disposed toward the patient or toward each other, "After all, not all sisters are the same."* And of course these days, in light of the AIDS epidemic, some people don't have sisters to rely on or compare.

I want to caution against putting Botswana and its forms of prognostication into some sort of evolutionary model in which, eventually, Batswana will become autonomous enough to take control over their own medical care and futures. There are several problems with fetishizing autonomy as progress, as some would do. First, there is a temporality to prognostic desire, even in places that privilege autonomy. As conditions deteriorate and the terminal phase of illness accelerates, patients often want less blunt information than they did in earlier phases of their treatment.[16] Second, deeming autonomy as progress implies a uniformity of desire by patients within a particular national culture and historical epoch. Yet there are people in present-day America who dislike the bluntness and abstractions of statistically based temporal prognostication and prefer the production of tacit knowledge, just as there were people in the past who abhorred the fictive dramas of tacit knowledge production, perhaps best exemplified in Tolstoy's classic novella *The Death of Ivan Ilyich*. David Rieff's extraordinary memoir of his mother Susan Sontag's death from cancer is instructive in this way.[17] For Sontag, the quintessential autonomous subject, hearing a terminal prognosis was simply unbearable. She fought against this both by submitting herself to extreme biotechnical interventions and by tacitly creating a socially enacted fictive drama of possible cure that foreclosed death talk. What Rieff's book makes clear is the tremendously social nature of Sontag's autonomy—something of which Batswana are already well aware. Third, autonomy, however important, is always deeply constrained by market forces that structure treatment options, and an obsession with autonomy as *the* ethical principle that matters in clinical discussions threatens to mask the political economy of therapeutic options in the language of choice.[18] Fourth, even Batswana who wish to know their terminal prognoses must still grapple with the potential toxicities of this knowledge in a world that actively recognizes the enormous potential for death to engender social rupture and discord. So, too, in America—social death threatens to precede biological death for the terminally ill.

American oncologists soften terminal prognoses and pronouncements of therapeutic futility by committing to their patients that they will be with them, palliating and caring for them even as they journey toward death.[19] In other sites in Africa, clinicians preferred to build up layers of tacit knowledge in patients, what Julian Harris, John Shao, and Jeremy Sugarman, in their work on cancer prognoses in Tanzania, call a "roundabout approach."[20] In this manner the doctor is able to gauge patient readiness and understanding, and to establish knowledge about the situation over time. Yet in PMH the rationing of bed-space prevents doctors and nurses from following a terminal prognosis with a definitive commitment to serve the patient, not to abandon her care and comfort even when specific treatments are no longer in the offing, despite the severity of suffering or the advocacy of relatives and staff. Nor is there time and space for the "roundabout" approach, given the pressures of the escalating cancer epidemic. This inability to commit to continued care for the patient necessarily shifts the ethics and possibilities of prognostication.

Autonomy cannot solve the problem presented by the shortage of beds. Nor can it solve the problem of therapeutic futility for patients with end-stage cancer. Nor can desperately ill Batswana care for themselves.

And so the type of paternalism practiced in PMH oncology works to distribute scarce resources in the face of ever-growing demand. Dr. P's authority is integral to the triage logic of the ward and therefore is carried as a burden by this oncologist who must do the unpleasant work of rationing care for the sick. Paternalism here also rationalizes the withholding of critical information from dying patients, distributing it instead to relatives, a form of communication that many Batswana endorse. Within the emerging post-ARV culture of technoscientific future-making brought by the upsurge in late-stage cancers, the power of decision making remains primarily in Dr. P's hands. He must decide when, amid the promise of new technology and the potent realities of a novel disease, to instruct relatives to give up and accept the inevitability of death.

Discussions with relatives, intended to provide a check on the nature of medical paternalism in the cancer ward, often end up reinforcing the differences in knowledge and power inherent to the clinical relationship. This is because the novelty of cancer works against meaningful communication. In PMH oncology, as in U.S. hospitals, prognostication around terminal illness occurred over time. The trajectories of dying usually unfolded in a series of discussions with relatives, intended to allow the prognosis to become clearer in stages. During "counseling sessions," some relatives remained silent, listening intently to Dr. P or to the nurse who was translating from English to Setswana, if such translation was necessary. The first of such conversations was often more positive, with relatives reassuring Dr. P that they knew he would try his best, and perhaps remarking that only God knows when someone will die. By the third or fourth such conversation, as therapies began to fail, many sat looking straight ahead, perhaps dabbing tears from the corners of their eyes. Relatives sometimes asked questions. A few had done preliminary research on the Internet; people came with widely divergent baselines of biomedical understanding. Many such conversations were necessarily brief, given the crush of work in the ward, and Dr. P's impatience. Relatives then tried to wedge them open, to instantiate the singularity of the life at hand.

In May 2009, Dikeledi lay dying in female cubicle A, bed 5. She was thirty-eight years old, and her cervical cancer was so advanced and aggressive that tumors had erupted all over her abdomen, like a rash. She was suffering mightily. One morning Dr. Z, the Congolese medical officer, drew blood from her inguinal veins, saying, "Sorry, mama, sorry,

sorry, mama." The pain was overwhelming, and she wept silently as I held her steady for the procedure, all the while rubbing her shoulders. In the afternoon Dr. P met with her older sister in the clinic office for "counseling" while a beautiful green and yellow bird sat watching us from the flame tree outside the window. "The message is short and unpleasant," he began. "The disease has spread all over her body . . . so she is going to die from this disease in the very near future. So we need to think about what we are going to do."* The sister inquired about treatment. "No, not about treatment," Dr. P continued, "but about where she is going to stay. She has had all the treatment. . . . So we have to prepare ourselves for the worst outcome. And there is no reason not to talk straight to you."* Her sister decided to "talk straight" back.

> "Being someone with a non-health perspective, I can tell she is deteriorating. She's got two kids. It is me and her, and we lost our mom a few years ago. You don't know her. She is on the soft side, my sister. And being sick, it can change a person, so she is not a self-centered kind of person, she has cause to complain."* Dr. P agreed. She does have hundreds of reasons to complain. Her sister continued, "I think she can tell, even now she wanted to come and hear what is to be said. But how long can she hang on? When I go there, she is going to want to know."*
>
> "No, everyone needs a little bit of hope—just a bit, so it is better she doesn't know, but with you, you must know. It is tough," Dr. P says. "But we have another problem—we need the bed."* "No. We've lost our mother, it is me and her. She is not in a condition to come home, even though I agree the situation in this ward is depressing." After some debate, they agree to put her in the queue for a bed in the private ward, for which the sister will pay a fee. We go back to the ward where Dikeledi is lying in her pale blue nightgown. Dr. P explains, "The disease has spread all over [your] body, and unfortunately there is no treatment we can give you right now. You have been blasted with too many treatments, and you need rest. We must wait."
>
> Dikeledi nods. "OK, so you cannot treat me now, but what about the pain?" So Dr. P increases her morphine. Her sister says, "Yes, but I have hope that you might feel better. I know, doctor, that you are trying your best." Dikeledi offers her part in this ritual: "Yes, I also have that hope, hope you will find a way to help me. I have faith you will help me." Her sister agrees: "Faith in God, so that God will help you." Dr. P, always the Marxist, cannot resist the moment: "I am not so sure God knows me!"* And the four

of us erupt in laughter. Dikeledi, though now bent over vomiting, is notice-ably more peaceful after this exercise in tacit prognostication.

At the heart of these complicated dynamics surrounding therapeu-tic futility for dying cancer patients lies an intangible—hope. In onco-logical counseling sessions with relatives and in clinical encounters with patients, long-standing biomedical and particularly oncological em-phases on "hope" mix with a social ethos among Batswana of commit-ment to an active present for the afflicted and also with an emergent biotechnical optimism among many who are now gaining experience with the power of ARVs. These sensibilities together produce a clinical encounter that further troubles the stakes and the contours of both the medical paternalism and the distributed autonomy I've described, and in turn the dynamics by which hope and futility are located and determined through acts of hospitalization.

The sociologist Shai Lavi, in his work on the history of euthanasia in America, describes the historical emergence of death as a technomedi-cal problem of hopelessness and pain. Beginning in the nineteenth cen-tury, as doctors began to take over from clergy at the deathbed, "the task of the physician was not merely to create a feeling of hope but to secure one based on the healing powers of medicine."[21] This emphasis on hope was what caused doctors to withhold terminal prognoses from patients until the emphasis on autonomy shifted practice in the United States. Yet even as autonomy has ushered in widespread disclosure of terminal prognoses, hope as a therapeutic method persists in wide-ranging forms, from heroic medicine, to terminal patient participation in phase I clinical trials, to the tremendous emphasis on pushing the cutting edge of medi-cal and bioscientific research. In Botswana, perched on the periphery of the oncological imagination, hope must find a different grounding.

Oncology as an international politicocultural practice and dynamic body of knowledge emphasizes "hope" as a vital force for orienting and animating biotechnical research, patient narratives, and practices of care.[22] For oncologists, researchers, fundraisers, and cancer patients, hope emerges as a mantra that discursively anchors the center of a vast and complicated enterprise. Oncology produces knowledge and uncer-tainty, therapy and futility constantly and simultaneously, and hope pro-vides much-needed ballast for well-meaning and sometimes desperate people. In the dark moments that shadow all cancer wards, hope that

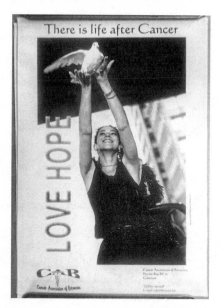

Cancer Association of Botswana poster promoting hope.

patients, knowledge, and techniques will improve is crucial to this often brutal and violent, if well-meaning, domain of technoscientific practice. Indeed, so much hope is wielded so often that it seems impossible that so little improvement has actually occurred in survival rates for many high-profile cancers such as breast cancers over the past century.[23] At its most cynical, hope and the repetition of its name provides a fig leaf for an enormous multibillion-dollar biotechnological industry. As Sarah Lochlann Jain cautions, our focus on the atomized hope of individuals distracts us from a broader oncological politics of publics living in a toxic and capitalistic world.[24] Botswana's position as an African nation that against all odds on the continent prioritizes universal healthcare and corporate capitalism simultaneously, and as a place where the cancer epidemic itself is in some part an outgrowth of a philanthropic project by Merck pharmaceuticals to extend the lives of those with HIV through the provision of antiretrovirals suggests a somewhat different, but no less compelling politics afoot.

Mothusi was not alone in arriving at PMH with relatives who expected and strongly advocated for therapeutic intervention for their patient. Dr. P was often met with pleas for action. Many families or individual patients came to their own conclusions about biomedical futility on the ward and refused disfiguring surgeries, or brought their patients home to die of their own initiative, to seek bongaka (Tswana medicine) or Christian healing prophesy, refusing further chemotherapeutic or other interventions. But many more pivoted around questions of futility and hope, insisting to Dr. P: "Can't you at least give him chemo?" "Please, just scan her!" "Put her in the machine and burn her!" "Please, please, doctor, can't you cut a hole in his throat so he can breathe?" "Feed him through a tube?" "Give her an IV?!" Such requests underscore the learning curve around biotechnical interventions, but they also indicate the extent to which hospitalization is becoming a method of hope, as Hirokazu Miyakazi would put it, for some Batswana.[25]

This stance surprised me at first. I had worked in Botswana in the 1990s, when most people I met were highly cynical about biomedicine.[26] For over a decade, people heard relentless messages about AIDS being a death sentence, then watched many people die ugly deaths. Now, though deaths continue, many are seeing their own bodies and those of their neighbors, coworkers, and relatives reconstituting—and the technologies that have produced such stunning reversals are at the hospital. Increasingly, one sees relatives pushing for more highly technologized interventions for the supposedly dying, and allowing a little bit of hope to seep into decisions to hospitalize.

Where American oncologists and their dying cancer patients might find hope in clinical trials, Dr. P could not. And when Mma Pula's daughter asked me how she, her own daughter, and her mother might all get into a clinical trial for their HIV, it was not to access cutting-edge therapies for Mma Pula's cervical cancer, but rather to facilitate free transportation and access to PMH where the morphine lay. Given the instability of knowledge in PMH oncology, Dr. P might still find hope in the clinical uncertainties that pervaded PMH and decide to work empirically with ample intellectual rationale for fulfilling the wishes of relatives. Meanwhile, for many Batswana cancer patients, hope was not so much for the progression of medical knowledge through research and experiment, but rather a political and economic hope that powerful modalities produced elsewhere, like oncology itself, would now be available to them as well.

Such hope by the broader community of patients, relatives, and clinical staff was not always misplaced. More than once in my time at PMH, I saw patients who were dying, whose relatives had been counseled, who were not expected to see the end of the week, rebound and recover in truly stunning ways. Such patients were particular favorites of the ward, and when they would return for follow-up visits, staff would slap them on the back or shake hands, saying to each other, "Remember him?" and "Look at her now—I almost don't recognize her!" And so the cycle of hope was an internally regenerative one, amid real uncertainties about how to manage the process of dying—socially, technologically, spatially, culturally, morally—so long as there was a bed available.

Changing Wards,
Further Improvisations

The cancer ward that I have described in this book no longer exists. A different oncology ward has taken its place. The sounds of vomiting, suctioning, and laughter continue, as do the smells of antiseptic, rot, and air freshener. Mma M is still ward matron, and a force for what Batswana call *botho* (humanity and care) in a crowded hospital. Patients still sit on the broken chair and exam table in the chemo room, tethered to the intravenous pole. Some patients are in remission. Some are cured. Plenty are dying. The cancer epidemic continues. But there is no crate of fruit in the office, and no one to slip Dintle a twenty-pula banknote each time she comes for her blood tests. No one is there to say, "This is a total disaster," repeatedly throughout the day. Dr. P is gone. In late 2009, after nearly a decade in exile, he completed his contract and returned home to Bulawayo. A tentative calm had come to that city, and Mpilo Hospital was busy rebuilding after the crisis years of 2006–8, when Robert Mugabe's government had brought Zimbabwe to the bloody brink of collapse.

A Chinese oncologist, Dr. X, sent on a three-year contract as part of a bilateral agreement between China and Botswana, has taken Dr. P's place in PMH oncology. Dr. K, the Zimbabwean radiation oncologist who worked alongside Dr. P at Mpilo in the 1990s, now comes two mornings a week to advise Dr. X and to help with the ever-growing volume of PMH cancer patients. But Dr. X has no cytology experience and no desire to sit at the microscope each evening. A crucial element of diagnosis was lost to Botswana when Dr. P returned to Zimbabwe, just as it had been lost to Zimbabwe when Dr. P crossed the border, in 2001, to open the PMH oncology ward.

Dr. P, Dr. K, PMH, and Mpilo Hospital are part of an uneven regional landscape that operates to some extent as a zero-sum game. It is a place where one hospital has brachytherapy, another has morphine, and another has an ear, nose, and throat specialist, but none has all three at once. In this region, too, "development" can be as much about repeatedly starting over as it is about methodically plodding forward.[1] When Dr. P first arrived at Mpilo, Zimbabwe was the best-case scenario for healthcare in the region. It was overcoming a colonial history of institutional racism and inequity by redirecting its abundant human resources and very good infrastructure. Yet all of these advantages, including most of the doctors and nurses, went away. In the late 1990s, Botswana's carefully planned path of healthcare development was overwhelmed by the epidemic of HIV/AIDS. PMH endured several years of extreme crisis, which included shutting down wards. What one sees in Mpilo and PMH are people—patients, nurses, doctors, technicians, relatives—simply trying to hold the pieces together. Such a context gives improvisation, cancer, and oncology a particular locality and meaning in the lives of southern African patients amid an escalating epidemic.

So cancer care continues at PMH, but its changed nature stands as a reminder that massive institutions, like "global health" or "oncology," occur on the ground through the work of specific individuals laboring in particular circumstances. It makes clear that the steady state of institutions in the region is a fragile one.

When Dr. P arrived at Mpilo Hospital in November of 2009, his first order of business was to restart the laboratory. Opening the door to the room where he had once spent so many thousands of hours, he felt as though he were entering a tomb. With the loss of staff and supplies, the laboratory had remained essentially dormant since he had left it, eight years earlier. After cleaning out the dust and debris, he hired a skilled laboratory technician he had worked with in the 1990s. Together they began to process several years of samples, which were sitting in formalin, waiting to be analyzed. Dr. P was now in semiretirement. As the only hematologist in Bulawayo, he was overseeing the care of a handful of private patients. But he was mainly committed to using his cytological skills and his clinical expertise to support the efforts of Dr. V, a young Zimbabwean doctor who was completing her specialty training in radiation oncology, and Dr. E, the Cuban oncologist who worked alongside her.

In September 2010 I flew to Zimbabwe to visit Dr. P and see how he was faring. Bulawayo, Zimbabwe's second largest city, looked tired and shabbier than I had ever seen it, but still beautiful. The famous jacaranda trees were poised to bloom. Mma S's women's club had organized a massive community effort to clean up and restore a large public park on the outskirts of Bulawayo, and we found families picnicking in the shade and chatting at the park café when we visited. There was petrol for sale, and the electrical power was on for most of the day, except for scheduled cuts that rotated neighborhoods (as in Gaborone in recent years). Presumably clean water was coming out of the taps, though after the cholera epidemic of 2008, many people thought it wise to boil the water just in case.

Bulawayo was still rebounding from its protracted economic decline over the 2000s and during the crisis years of 2006–8, when the Zimbabwean economy collapsed in a spiral of hyperinflation, and basic services dried up, replaced by escalating political violence. By September 2010, however, when I arrived, the situation had stabilized amid widespread poverty. Tendai Biti, the finance minister of the new coalition government, had abandoned the Zimbabwean currency, allowing people to use U.S. dollars, South African rand, and Botswana pula as hard currency in their daily transactions, which had steadied matters. Women were carefully washing the precious, rapidly circulating dollar bills and hanging them on clothespins to dry. Goods had returned to the markets, and petrol to the filling stations, though there was little cash in most pockets. No one knew how long the stability would last, or if violence and collapse would return, but for the meanwhile people in Bulawayo were trying to rebuild.

Mpilo, the main public hospital for Bulawayo, had staggered through its own cycles of degradation and collapse. Mpilo's demise was a long time in the making. Zimbabwe's planned transition from a racially segregated health service prioritizing clinical care to a minority white population, to one that prioritized both primary care for the majority black population and expanded access to sophisticated tertiary care, while admirable, proved difficult. Successes were notable, but resisting the trend of widespread privatization of public health in Africa proved impossible.[2] In the late 1980s and early 1990s, even as the Botswana government was expanding primary care and sending some of the few cancer patients to Mpilo, doctors and nurses were starting to leave Zimbabwe for Botswana and South Africa. IMF-led economic structural adjustment was undermining salaries, even as it was failing to ameliorate the problem of importing necessary medical supplies and technologies. Private healthcare began to thrive as public patients faced greater vulnerabilities.[3] When Dr. P left Zimbabwe in 2001, he was part of a mass exodus of experienced medical staff who had come to find clinical, political, and economic conditions uncertain and troubling. The failure of Zimbabwe's program of social medicine would carry tremendous costs for Zimbabwean patients, including those with cancer.

While I was sitting in PMH oncology witnessing a system of universal care (warts and all), patients in Zimbabwe and their caregivers were witnessing the privatization and ultimate failure of biomedical services. By 2006, most doctors, nurses, and technicians had left the country, and those who remained often waited months for overdue paychecks, the value of which was already outstripped by hyperinflation. Striking public-sector doctors in 2007 claimed to be "among the lowest paid professionals in Zimbabwe, earning less than the equivalent of $1 per day at the black market exchange rate."[4] Uncollected bodies were left piled high in the hospital morgue, as relatives were unable to pay transport and burial costs, and Mpilo Hospital went weeks at a time without running water. Basic supplies—including intravenous fluids, plaster of Paris, glucose sticks, antiseptic, bandages, catheter bags, and syringes—went out of stock, as did crucial drugs, while equipment such as dialysis machines lay in disrepair in what was once, by all accounts, an excellent hospital.[5] Some people shared stories of profound physical agony and deaths born of the near total lack of medicines, sutures, and bandages. Those few doctors and nurses who remained were forced to make terrible choices as they improvised in impossible circumstances. Some went to great lengths to help patients, but I also heard stories of crass exploitation.

For the time being, it seemed the worst was over. But Mpilo was only a shadow of its former self. It was hard to imagine that this was once the place Botswana sent some of its most complicated medical cases, including many cancer patients. Amid the rebuilding, Mpilo staff and patients were improvising on many levels. One day I attended the morning meeting for the medical ward at Mpilo, just as I had many times at PMH. Unlike at PMH, where we sat crowded in a small cement room attached to the medical ward, at Mpilo we gathered around a large seminar table in a medical library lined with bookshelves, which were filled with old medical journals and above which hung portraits of great white doctors past. Dr. D, a young Zimbabwean medical officer, presented the case for discussion. The case hinged on a differential diagnosis of toxoplasmosis, cytomegalovirus, non-Hodgkin's lymphoma with central nervous system involvement, cryptococcus, and one or two other possibilities.[6] Dr. D explained that given the lack of laboratory capacity to support possible diagnostic tests at present, he would suspect toxoplasmosis and proceed accordingly. Dr. P questioned this decision, then provided some epidemiological data from Botswana that suggested other potential problems were not so easily discounted. But Dr. D explained that they always went with toxoplasmosis, in large part because it was the only condition on the list that they could treat with a drug the hospital stocked. The staff then discussed how they would proceed with such a case *if* their imaging and laboratory technologies were available and *if* an array of drugs and other therapeutic interventions were present. In other words, the doctors at Mpilo Hospital were producing knowledge on two levels simultaneously. One was intended to maintain their professional expertise for a possible future in a fully functioning Mpilo, and the other to sharpen their empirical skills for the here and now, which meant a continual recalibration of diagnostic ability, therapeutic supply, and epidemiological knowledge.

Inside the oncology clinic, Dr. K's nameplate was still on the office door. It had been seven years since he had left Mpilo for Botswana; perhaps now that his replacement, Dr. V, had finally arrived, there would be cause to change the nameplate. The men's medical ward looked fairly calm and well organized compared to its counterpart at PMH. In the oncology clinic, while receiving chemo, patients sat on lounge chairs watching reruns of Barney Miller on a television suspended from the wall in a spacious room. The waiting line was shorter than at PMH, and Mpilo had two oncologists working in the clinic, supported by a medical officer. The hospital had a whole radiotherapy setup, with a linear accelerator, a cobalt 60 unit (now decommissioned), and a brachytherapy facility for internal radiation. There was even a sign for a department of nuclear medicine, though it was long since defunct.

At first glance I was impressed by how tidy (despite the broken toilets and missing floor tiles), how relatively orderly Mpilo seemed compared to PMH. I saw no patients lying on the floors. The oncologists each saw no more than fifteen outpatients a day and had no ward to manage (in fact, Mpilo oncology had no inpatients at all). Dr. V had time to counsel patients, to listen to their anxieties, to encourage them, to explain, and she was quite thoughtful about this aspect of her work. What I came to understand, however, was that this orderliness came at a terrible price. The relative calm in Mpilo oncology did not mean that somehow Zimbabwe had escaped Botswana's escalating cancer epidemic, nor that well-planned resources meant a more humane standard of care. It only meant that, like in most of Africa (but unlike in Botswana), cancer medicine here was now essentially privatized, and therefore unobtainable for the vast majority of patients. It also suggested that broken equipment, uneven staffing, and uncertain supplies were so entrenched that many families were uncertain whether to invest in highly improvised oncology.

What does privatization mean in practice? One morning, Dr. V and I crossed the clinic hall, at the request of Dr. E, to talk to the family of an elderly man with advanced prostate cancer. The patient was sitting awkwardly, gripping the white plastic chair. With metastases boring into his bones, he was in tremendous pain, but there was no morphine or codeine in stock in the hospital pharmacy. Nor was either drug available at the private pharmacies in the city. Dr. V knew this firsthand, as she had been unable to secure pain medication for her cousin, who had died of cancer the previous week, until she had sent a relative to the central hospital in Harare, where morphine was suddenly, temporarily, in stock. As the day progressed, a twenty-one-year-old woman whose knee was destroyed from KS arrived with her brother. Her mother waited in the hall. Dr. V handed prescriptions to the brother, who then had to take a taxi-bus to a pharmacy in town, buy the chemotherapy drugs, and bring them back to Mpilo for injection. Some patients could afford only one or two out of three of their chemotherapy drugs, and so were not taking the standard course. We crisscrossed between the clinic and the antiquated brachytherapy machine, to which women with cervical cancer were connected one by one for their treatment.

Then, into the clinic walked a thin woman in her late thirties wearing a well-worn dress and long cardigan. She was a teacher at a local school. In 2006 she had undergone a lumpectomy at a private hospital in Bulawayo, paid for by the insurance her husband's job provided. Her doctor wrote her a prescription for tamoxifen. Shortly thereafter, her doctor, like so many other medical professionals, felt compelled to leave Zimbabwe. At the time of her lumpectomy, there was no oncologist in Bulawayo, and the radiotherapy machines were not working. So she did not undergo the adjuvant radiation that would have been part of the standard of care for her case. She had been managing to refill the tamoxifen since then, through a pharmacist she knew. But now that there was an oncologist in Bulawayo again, the pharmacist had urged her to come to Mpilo for a check-up. So here she was. She was nervous. She had reason to be.

With some effort and encouragement, she got up on the table and removed her bra. Dr. V found a hard node in her armpit. When the patient dressed and returned to her chair, Dr. V proceeded gingerly: "You have done very, very well for four years." But already the patient was crying. She knew what was coming. "We need to take a biopsy, a small piece of that hard thing under your arm. You have done so well and been so committed in taking your tamoxifen. But tamoxifen is not necessarily enough to control cancer. Usually we would have given you radiotherapy after the surgery, but it wasn't available at that time. So we need a biopsy to see. If this is the same cancer back, then, well, we know what to do. If it isn't, it is more difficult to decide."

Dr. V was in a difficult situation. There were no notes from the surgeon, who already had operated under challenging circumstances. There was no histology report in the patient's file either, though the tissue sample was presumably stored in Harare. But it would be difficult to trace. Then it turned out the patient was in an even more difficult situation. Her husband had lost his job, which had been their source of Medical Aid (insurance). She could not afford surgery. She was not alone in this situation. Earlier that morning, I had visited the 250-bed private hospital where she had undergone her original surgery, and there were only a handful of inpatients listed on the board. Meanwhile, Mpilo was without a general surgeon on staff and soon would close its general surgery practice entirely.[7]

Dr. V said, "Look, I cannot lie to you. This is going to be very hard. The wait for public patients is a three-month list right now, and then something inevitably breaks in the operating theater, the wait gets longer, people wind up pushed down the list, etcetera. General surgery is very hard right now, and you would need to get it done at the private hospital, because there is no general surgeon at Mpilo right now." The patient knew she could not afford it. She began to cry again. Then Dr. V remembered that Dr. P was now back at Mpilo and could do a needle biopsy. "This is good. It will not cost, and hopefully it will yield answers right away."

The next day Dr. P read the slide and learned it was indeed malignant, so the patient paid a small fee to have the original biopsy sample retested in Harare and a report sent. Progress was made, but a recurrence is every breast cancer patient's worst fear. The patient's tears, her frustration pointed backward to a bleak past of fleeing surgeons, absent oncologists, broken machines, and lost jobs, as well as forward to a difficult future, of costly and distressing surgery and chemotherapy, amid myriad uncertainties. But her arrival in Mpilo that day also marked a new present: a time when after a long hiatus there was once again a young, energetic, and committed radiation oncologist, and once again an experienced hematologist-oncologist-cytologist making diagnoses, a time where care once again seemed possible.

This book has seen the PMH oncology ward as a microcosm, an instantiation of global health, of southern African history, of cancer, of Botswana in miniature. But the PMH oncology ward, as part of a government program of universal care, is only one possibility for an African cancer ward. Another possibility lies in its Mpilo counterpart. Their entangled pasts; their reversal of fortune; the cyclical movement of clinical staff, patients, knowledge, and goods across the Botswana-Zimbabwe border; their current contrasts; and the futures to which they point underscore the fragility of institutions in a region with a long history of sudden reversals. Against this context of fragility, improvising medicine, like cancer itself, is a daily imperative.

An asterisk by quoted speech indicates that I am certain I have the words verbatim.

PREFACE

1 Wainana, "How to Write about Africa."
2 Comaroff, "The Diseased Heart of Africa."
3 Wainana, "How to Write about Africa."

ONE ⚕ THE OTHER CANCER WARD

1 Nyangabwe patients sometimes come to PMH on referral, either to be cared for during radiotherapy (in which case they are driven each day to GPH for time in the radiation machine) or for clinical consultation, but PMH patients do not go to Nyangabwe, unless they relocate north.
2 The diamond industry, Debswana, maintains two hospitals; the Botswana Defense Force (the national military) maintains another; and there is a private hospital in Gaborone, another in the final stages of construction, and many private clinics and doctor's offices for those with health insurance, deep pockets, or enough desperation or frustration with the public system that they are willing to pay for care.
3 Wendland, *A Heart for the Work.*
4 Kleinman and Hanna, "Catastrophe, Caregiving and Today's Biomedicine"; Theresa Brown, *Critical Care.*
5 Garcia, *The Pastoral Clinic,* 50. See also Tronto, *Moral Boundaries.*
6 Livingston, *Debility and the Moral Imagination in Botswana;* Biehl, *Vita;* Garcia, *The Pastoral Clinic.*
7 I am especially grateful to Vinh-Kim Nguyen for helping me to sort out this last point.
8 On oncological hope, see Good, Good, Schaffer, and Lind, "American On-

cology and the Discourse of Hope"; Ehrenreich, "Pathologies of Hope"; Jain, "The Mortality Effect." On the African ethic of continuous effort, see Whyte, *Questioning Misfortune*; Langwick, *Bodies, Politics, and African Healing*; Klaits, *Death in a Church of Life*; Geissler and Prince, *The Land Is Dying*.

9 Parkin, Sitas, Chirenje, Stein, Abratt, and Waibinga, "Part 1: Cancer in Indigenous Africans," 683.

10 Ngoma, "World Health Organization Cancer Priorities in Developing Countries," viii9.

11 Farmer et al., "Expansion of Cancer Care and Control in Countries of Low and Middle Income"; Travis, "Cancer in Africa"; Morris, "Cancer?"; Lingwood et al., "The Challenge of Cancer Control in Africa"; Sloan and Gelband, *Cancer Control Opportunities in Low- and Middle-Income Countries*; Ngoma, "World Health Organization Cancer Priorities in Developing Countries"; Boyle et al., "Editorial."

12 Cytology is a method of diagnosing disease by examining cellular morphology. In PMH oncology, Dr. P extracts lymphatic or other fluid (through a process called a fine-needle aspiration or, less frequently, a bone-marrow aspiration or even a bone-marrow biopsy) and then presses the cells onto slides. These cells are stained, and he then examines them under a microscope, searching the slides for the presence of particular cellular structures that suggest what type of malignancy, if any, is present. With histology (or histopathology), a biopsy — a surgical sample of presumably diseased tissue — is processed into slices, placed on slides, stained, and then given to a pathologist, who examines the structures of the tissue sample under the microscope to identify any malignancy.

13 Boyle and Levin, *World Cancer Report 2008*, 15–16.

14 Songolo, Chokuonga, Motlogi, and Mogorsakgomo, *Botswana National Cancer Registry Report, 1986–2004*, 15.

15 Parkin, Sitas, Chirenje, Stein, Abratt, and Waibinga, "Part 1: Cancer in Indigenous Africans," 684.

16 In other words, since cancer risks increase with age, age-standardization statistically realigns both southern Africa's youth-heavy age pyramid and North America's demographic bloat of aging baby-boomers to allow for comparisons across age cohorts, rather than across aggregate populations.

17 Aronowitz, "The Converged Experience of Risk and Disease."

18 Parkin, Bray, Ferlay, and Pisani, "Global Cancer Statistics, 2002," 82, table 3.

19 Parkin, Sitas, Chirenje, Stein, Abratt, and Waibinga, "Part 1: Cancer in Indigenous Africans," 683.

20 Feigal and Black, "Cancer and AIDS"; Travis, "Cancer in Africa." Through the past decade, CD4 cell counts have been used to triage patients in need of ARVs. The program in Botswana began by starting patients on treatment if their CD4 count was 200 or below, or if they had an AIDS indicator illness. Eventually, the cutoff point was raised to 250, then to 300. In practice, this requires that people be tested before they are symptomatic and that the CD4 machines be in working condition (they break down regularly). In other countries, where the ARV programs are patched together among various NGO and government

initiatives, there are still significant problems of access, even for those with low counts. Over time we can hope (but not necessarily expect) that ARV programs develop to the point where most patients are initiated on antiretrovirals while their CD4 counts are still high enough to help them avoid such cancers, as has happened in the United States. But even if African AIDS programs can overcome the infrastructural, financial, and other obstacles to pursue such a policy, experience in the United States has shown that the cancer problem will likely shift shape rather than simply disappear. In the United States, while ARVs have resulted in a crucial reduction in the numbers of HIV-positive patients with AIDS-defining cancers, over time there has also been a rise in those with non-AIDS-defining cancers. Shiels et al., "Cancer Burden in the HIV-Infected Population in the United States."

21 Merriweather, *Desert Doctor Remembers*, 79.

22 Johnson, "The Cases of Cancer Seen at a Botswana Hospital 1968–1972."

23 Macrae and Cook, "A Retrospective Study of the Cancer Patterns among Hospital In-Patients in Botswana, 1960–72."

24 Livingston, "AIDS as Chronic Illness."

25 Good, "The Biotechnical Embrace." See also Keirns, "Dying of a Treatable Disease."

26 Durham and Klaits, "Funerals and the Public Space of Sentiment in Botswana"; Klaits, *Death in a Church of Life*; Dow and Essex, *Saturday Is for Funerals*; Livingston, *Debility and the Moral Imagination in Botswana*; Dahl, "Left Behind?"; Ngwenya and Butale, "HIV/AIDS, Intra-family Resource Capacity and Home Care in Maun"; Heald, "It's Never as Easy as ABC."

27 Creek et al., "Successful Introduction of Routine Opt-Out HIV Testing in Antenatal Care in Botswana"; Bussmann et al., "Five-Year Outcomes of Initial Patients Treated in Botswana's National Antiretroviral Treatment Program"; Ramiah and Reich, "Building Effective Public-Private Partnerships." See also Brada, "Botswana as a Living Experiment."

28 Carpenter, "The Social Practice of HIV Drug Therapy in Botswana, 2002–2004."

29 Whyte, Whyte, Meinart, and Kyaddondo, "Treating AIDS"; Mulemi, "Coping with Cancer and Adversity."

30 For more on the privatization of healthcare in Africa, see Turshen, *Privatizing Health Services in Africa*; Nguyen, "Government by Exception."

31 Nyati-Ramahobo, "From a Phone Call to the High Court"; Werbner, "Challenging Minorities, Differences, and Tribal Citizenship in Botswana"; Solway, "Human Rights and NGO 'Wrongs'"; Nyamnjoh, *Insiders and Outsiders*; Van Allen, "'Bad Future Things' and Liberatory Moments."

32 Central Intelligence Agency, *The World Fact Book, 2010*, accessed 28 September 2010.

33 Livingston, "Suicide, Risk, and Investment in the Heart of the African Miracle."

34 "Botswana: Bleak Outlook for Future AIDS Funding," accessed 27 February 2012.

35 The best analysis of Botswana's place within the imaginary problem space of Global Health is Brada, "'Not *Here*.'"

36 Bosk, *Forgive and Remember*; Kohn, Corrigan, and Donaldson, *To Err Is Human*.

37 I also performed ethnographic and historical research on debility in Botswana in 1996, 1997, and 1998–1999. The results were published in Livingston, *Debility and the Moral Imagination in Botswana*.

38 This research was approved by three Institutional Review Boards: Rutgers University, Protocol # 01–355 M, "Pain and Laughter: A History of Sentience in Botswana"; Ministry of Health, Republic of Botswana, Reference No: PPME-13/18/1 Vol 1 (224), "Pain: A History of Sentience in Botswana"; and the Ethics Panel of Princess Marina Hospital, Gaborone, Botswana.

39 Van der Geest and Finkler, "Hospital Ethnography"; Wind, "Negotiated Interactive Observation"; Mulemi, "Patients' Perspectives on Hospitalization"; Long, Hunter, and Van der Geest, "Introduction"; Finkler, Hunter, and Idema, "What Is Going On?"

40 Van der Geest and Kaja Finkler, "Hospital Ethnography." For excellent examples, see Kaufman, *And a Time to Die*; Rouse, *Uncertain Suffering*; Lock, *Twice Dead*.

41 I thank Seth Koven greatly for helping me think through the question of voice and epistemology.

42 By contrast, for an excellent patient-centered ethnography, see Mulemi, "Coping with Cancer and Adversity."

43 Ed Cohen, personal communication. See also Rachel Prentice's wonderful new book on embodied surgeons, *Bodies of Information*.

TWO ⚭ NEOPLASTIC AFRICA

1 World Health Organization, "Cholera in Zimbabwe," accessed 26 October 2009.

2 On xenophobia in Botswana, see Nyamnjoh, *Insiders and Outsiders*.

3 Farmer et al., "Expansion of Cancer Care and Control in Countries of Low and Middle Income."

4 The Summers memo of 12 December 1991, when he was vice president and chief economist of the World Bank, has been excerpted and reproduced on numerous websites, including http://www.jacksonprogressive.com, http://www.whirledbank.org, and http://www.mindfully.org.

5 Hunger is an extremely pressing problem, one that greatly complicates ARV provision. See, for example, Kalofonos, "All I Eat Is ARVs."

6 Stewart and Kleihues, *World Cancer Report*, 281–82.

7 Okeke, *Divining without Seeds*.

8 "Poverty Blamed for Blacks High Cancer Rate," *New York Times*, 17 April 1991; Wailoo, *How Cancer Crossed the Color Line*; Hecht, "Africa and the Nuclear World"; Hecht, *Uranium from Africa and the Power of Nuclear Things*.

9 There is an extensive literature on these issues in Africa: Packard, "The Healthy Reserve and the Dressed Native"; Comaroff, "The Diseased Heart of Africa"; Vaughan, *Curing Their Ills*. And, of course, see Fabian, *Time and the Other*.

10 Livingston, *Debility and the Moral Imagination*, chap. 4.

11 Nicholas B. King, "Security, Disease, Commerce"; Lakoff, "Two Regimes of Global Health"; Lakoff, "The Generic Biothreat."

12 Braun and Phoun, "HPV Vaccination Campaigns."

13 Stewart and Kleihues, *World Cancer Report*, 61.

14 Iliffe, *East African Doctors*, 142–43. See, for example, Burkitt and Kyalwazi, "Spontaneous Remission of African lymphoma"; Olweny, Toya, Katongole-Mbidde, Mugerwa, Kyalwazi, and Cohen, "Treatment of Hepatocellular Carcinoma with Adriamycin"; Vogel, Templeton, Templeton, Taylor, and Kyalwazi, "Treatment of Kaposi's Sarcoma with Actinomycin-D and Cyclophosphamide"; Taylor, Templeton, Vogel, Ziegler, and Kyalwazi, "Kaposi's Sarcoma in Uganda"; Ziegler, Cohen, Morrow, Kyalwazi, and Carbone, "Immunologic Studies in Burkitt's Lymphoma."

15 Carcinogenesis is complex and in many cases poorly understood, and I do not argue that these viruses in and of themselves *cause* cancers. Instead, it makes more sense to understand them as necessary, but not sufficient causes in many cases.

16 This history is outlined by the founding director of IARC in Higginson, "From Geographic Pathology to Environmental Carcinogenesis."

17 Higginson, "The International Agency for Research on Cancer," 80.

18 Ibid., 83.

19 And it was a paradigm in turn fostered by research into African cancers. See Maclean, "Nigeria 1956–65." I thank Iruka Okeke for bringing this to my attention.

20 Culliton, "Cancer," 1111.

21 Ibid.

22 Mukherjee, *The Emperor of All Maladies*, 357.

23 Proctor, *Cancer Wars*; Wailoo and Pemberton, *The Troubled Dream of Genetic Medicine*.

24 The Statute of the IAEA, Article II (Objectives), http://iaea.org/About/statute.html, accessed 27 February 2012.

25 Durosinmi-Etti, Nofal, and Mahfouz, "Radiotherapy in Africa," 24, 25.

26 Williams and O'Connor, "Introduction."

27 The Uganda Cancer Institute had grown out of a lymphoma treatment center at Mulago Hospital—initially funded, in the late 1960s, by the U.S. National Institute of Health—and was a site of American scientific collaboration in the early 1970s.

28 Williams, O'Connor, De-The, and Johnson, *Virus-Associated Cancers in Africa*, xxv–xxvi.

29 In the late 1980s and early 1990s there was clinical research and interest in AIDS-related malignancies, particularly KS and lymphoma, among U.S.-based researchers, but cases of cancer began to decline after the introduction of protease inhibitors in the mid-1990s. A greater flurry of work on AIDS-related malignancies (particularly non-Hodgkin's lymphoma, HPV-related genital cancers, and KS), including treatment recommendations, followed in the

late 1990s and early 2000s. See, for example, several of the articles collected in Feigal, Levine, and Biggar, AIDS-Related Cancers and Their Treatment. In 1995 the National Cancer Institute established the AIDS Malignancy Consortium (AMC), with fifteen primary clinical trials sites, to develop therapeutic protocols for AIDS-related cancers. Yet the AMC project was short-lived and was not re-funded when its grant expired, in 2004. For a brief overview of the AMC, see Shouten, "The Rise and Fall of the AIDS Malignancy Consortium."

30 Even such an astute critic of the cancer industrial complex as the historian of science Robert Proctor was able to claim in 1995, "It is probably fair to say that undue attention has been given to this particular collection of agents [viruses]. The same could be said for infectious agents more generally" (Cancer Wars, 14).

31 This is not to suggest that cancer was thought to be directly related to affluence. Scrotal cancers had long been associated with chimney sweeps, and mesothelioma with asbestos workers, for example. Rather it was associated with that problematic term modernity.

32 Fabian, Time and the Other.

33 See Packard, "Visions of Postwar Health and Development and Their Impact on Public Health Interventions in the Developing World"; Nicholas B. King, "Security, Disease, Commerce."

34 Turshen, Privatizing Health Services in Africa.

35 Gerrets, "Globalizing International Health"; Brada, "Botswana as a Living Experiment."

36 These changes are very complicated dynamics that incorporate dynamic legal and market structures accompanying the rise of the World Trade Organization, and attendant shifts in intellectual property rights. See Peterson, "On the Monopoly"; Biehl, "The Activist State"; Biehl, "Pharmaceuticalization."

37 Whyte, Whyte, Meinart, and Kyaddondo, "Treating AIDS"; Nguyen, The Republic of Therapy.

38 Biehl, "Pharmaceuticalization," 1093.

39 Ecks, "Global Pharmaceutical Markets and Corporate Citizenship," 172.

40 Ibid.

41 Biehl, "Pharmaceuticalization."

42 The appeal of the STD for making African health intelligible is long-standing. See Packard and Epstein, "Epidemiologists, Social Scientists and the Structure of Medical Research on AIDS in Africa"; Musisi, "The Politics of Perception or Perception as Politics?"; Vaughan, "Syphilis and Sexuality: The Limits of Colonial Medical Power," "Syphilis in the Uganda Protectorate," "Syphilis in Uganda"; Kark, "The Social Pathology of Syphilis in Africans"; Caldwell, Caldwell, and Quiggin, "The Social Context of AIDS in Sub-Saharan Africa"; Heald, "The Power of Sex"; Hunt, A Nervous State.

43 For a discussion of the challenges of screening through pap smear and colposcopy in these settings versus the new visual inspection with acetic acid ("see and treat"), see Denny, Quinn, and Sankaranarayanan, "Screening for Cervical Cancer in Developing Countries."

44 Ramogola-Masire, "Cervical Cancer, HIV and the HPV Vaccine in Botswana."

45 Livingston, Wailoo, and Cooper, "HPV Skepticism and Vaccination as Governance."

46 Sahasrabuddhe, "Prevalence and Distribution of HPV Genotypes among HIV-Infected Women in Zambia"; Wall et al., "Cervical Human Papillomavirus Infection and Squamous Intraepithelial Lesions in Rural Gambia, West Africa." See also Muñoz et al., "Epidemiological Classification of Human Papillomavirus Types Associated with Cervical Cancer."

47 McKenzie, Kobetz, Hnatyszyn, Twiggs, and Lucci, "Women with HIV Are More Commonly Infected with Non-16 and -18 High-Risk HPV Types," 573.

48 Louie, de Sanjose, and Mayaud, "Epidemiology and Prevention of Human Papillomavirus and Cervical Cancer in Sub-Saharan Africa."

49 McKenzie, Kobetz, Hnatyszyn, Twiggs, and Lucci, "Women with HIV Are More Commonly Infected with Non-16 and -18 High-Risk HPV Types," 573.

50 Haug, "Human Papillomavirus Vaccination."

51 I am grateful to Robby Aronowitz for this point.

52 Pettypiece, "Global," accessed 7 November 2009.

53 Livingston, *Debility and the Moral Imagination in Botswana*; Schapera, *Migrant Labour and Tribal Life*.

54 Packard, *White Plague, Black Labor*; Hunter, *Love in the Time of AIDS*; Fassin, *When Bodies Remember*.

55 Radon daughters are short-lived radioactive decay atoms that can attach to dust particles and produce ionizing radiation damage in the lung.

56 Engels et al., "Tuberculosis and Subsequent Risk of Lung Cancer in Xuanwei, China."

57 See, for example, Markowtiz and Rosner, *Deceit and Denial*; Rosner and Markowitz, *Deadly Dust, Silicosis and the Struggle for Workers' Health*; Warren, *Brush with Death*; Gabrielle Hecht, "Hopes for the Radiated Body."

58 African miners were not allowed to form unions in South Africa until the 1980s, and Africans were disenfranchised in South Africa until 1994, in South West Africa (now Namibia) until 1990, and in Southern Rhodesia (now Zimbabwe) until 1980.

59 Packard, *White Plague, Black Labor*; McCulloch, *Asbestos Blues*.

60 Hecht, "Africa and the Nuclear World."

61 Ibid., 791.

62 McCulloch, *Asbestos Blues*; Braun, "Structuring Silence"; Braun and Kisting, "Asbestos-Related Disease in South Africa."

63 Braun, "Structuring Silence," 59.

64 Milmo, "Dumped in Africa," accessed 9 October 2009; Abdullahi, "'Toxic Waste' behind Somali Piracy," accessed 9 October 2009. See, for example, *Toxic Exports*, Jennifer Clapp's excellent book on the subject; and Pellow, *Resisting Global Toxics*.

65 Brandt, *The Cigarette Century*, chap. 13; Sussman et al., "Tobacco Control in Developing Countries."

66 On China, see, for example, Kohrman and Shuiyuan, "Anthropology in China's Health Promotion and Tobacco."

67 World Health Organization, *Tobacco Atlas 2002*, accessed 14 February 2011. It is unclear to me how these numbers are generated, what differences there may be between urban and rural populations, how heavily such consumers smoke, and so on.

68 For example, total African cigarette consumption in 1995 was 131,181 million cigarettes. By 2000, the figure stood at 212,788 million, a nearly 40 percent increase in a half decade (Guindon and Boscar, *Past, Current, and Future Trends in Tobacco Use*).

69 Sasco, "From the International Union Against Cancer: Africa," 281.

70 Brandt, *The Cigarette Century*, 486.

THREE ◊ CREATING AND EMBEDDING CANCER

1 For the best extended discussion of this history, see Aronowitz, *Unnatural History*.

2 There is only one site I know of for mammography in Botswana. It is in a private radiography practice in a shopping mall in Gaborone. In all my time at PMH oncology, I saw only two women who went for mammography. Both times, Dr. P recognized that they had the resources to pay out of pocket for this imaging procedure before he suggested it. Both were postmastectomy breast cancer patients, who were getting a mammogram to screen their remaining breast.

3 Aronowitz, *Unnatural History*; Lock, "Breast Cancer"; Langwick, "Devils, Parasites, and Fierce Needles"; Langwick, *Bodies, Politics, and African Healing*; Michelle Murphy, *Sick Building Syndrome and the Politics of Uncertainty*; Mol, *The Body Multiple*.

4 And, of course, we have come to realize that, for example, not all prostate cancers within a given population will respond in equal fashion to particular therapies, nor will they result in identical or uniform disease trajectories. There is a tremendous amount of idiosyncrasy in the experience and expression of disease. Thus, even within a uniform infrastructural field, cancer raises basic questions of ontology.

5 It is not my intention to criticize the Cancer Association of Botswana, which is doing important work. In 2011, they launched a website that appears to be much better thought out than their earlier posters and pamphlets in how it presents information about cancer in Botswana.

6 See Biehl, "Pharmaceuticalization."

7 Readers in the United States will recognize this referral structure as similar to a health maintenance organization (HMO).

8 This is beginning to change, but very slowly. In 2008 I accompanied Dr. P on a trip organized by the ministry of health, which sends specialists of various types to the primary hospitals to help train clinical staff and sometimes see patients. On this occasion, we took a small plane to a remote primary hospital in the

Kalahari, where Dr. P gave a PowerPoint presentation on breast cancer meant to help clinical staff identify and refer patients.

9 This long quote is verbatim speech from an interview I conducted, tape recorded, and transcribed (recording in my possession).

10 This, too, is starting to change. When I returned to the PMH oncology ward in May 2009 after a ten-month absence, for the first time since I had begun my ethnographic work in the ward, Dr. P had a full staff of medical officers, and an oncologist had recently arrived from China to join him. At the same time, patient volume had only increased, so while Dr. P now worked only one weekend a month, otherwise enjoying five-day weeks, he still regularly put in long days.

11 In some ways we see here the opposite situation from that described in *The Body Multiple* by Annemarie Mol, who examines processes of coordination between different domains of the hospital in creating the patient and the disease.

12 In Setswana discussions about illness, people usually refer to the part of their body that is ailing. "I am ill. What is wrong? *Leteka* (waist), or *sefuba* (chest)." This is, in part, because Setswana illness categories can pathologize social relationships, so calling attention to a diagnosis means pointing to tensions within a family (a speech act that in itself can cause tensions). While public-health campaigns urge Batswana to discuss HIV openly, in the interest of doing away with its exceptional status, the public use of such an illness category itself would be somewhat exceptional. There are exceptions, of course, and some biomedical categories have entered into common use, like the terms *sugar diabetes* or *flu*.

13 Both are chemotherapy drugs.

14 I call this "metropolitan" knowledge, but my use of this shorthand term does not necessarily mean it was built through American, Japanese, or Western European bodies. As Adriana Petryna shows in *When Experiments Travel*, cancer-drug trials are increasingly being outsourced to places like Eastern Europe, Brazil, Argentina, and so on.

15 In the late 1980s and early 1990s there was clinical research and interest in AIDS-related malignancies, particularly KS and lymphoma among U.S.-based researchers, but cases of cancer began to decline after the introduction of protease inhibitors in the mid-1990s. A greater flurry of work on AIDS-related malignancies (particularly non-Hodgkin's lymphoma, HPV-related genital cancers, and KS), including treatment recommendations, followed in the late 1990s and early 2000s. See, for example, several of the articles collected in Feigal, Levine, and Biggar, *AIDS-Related Cancers and Their Treatment*. But the therapeutic guidance in this volume ranges from pronouncements of the difficulties of treating cervical cancer in HIV-positive individuals, to discussions of cytokines, which are not relevant to the PMH context. In 1995 the National Cancer Institute established the AIDS Malignancy Consortium (AMC) with fifteen main clinical trials sites to develop therapeutic protocols for AIDS-related cancers. But while the AMC focused on KS, lymphoma, and HPV, in Botswana

there are also high rates of head and neck tumors associated with HIV, as well as many other patients suffering from breast, lung, esophageal, leukemia, bone, and other cancers who happen to have HIV co-infection. For a brief overview of the AMC to 2003, see Shouten, "The Rise and Fall of the AIDS Malignancy Consortium." More recently, the AMC has begun research on non-AIDS-defining cancers and has a new mandate to "expand their capacity to conduct trials in Africa." National Cancer Institute, Office of HIV and AIDS Malignancy, "AIDS Malignancy Consortium," accessed 26 July 2011.

16 Similarly, it is hard to make room for the "local biology" of Botswana's HIV-related cancer within the AIDS establishment. International protocols for HIV management and funding come from places like the United States. This means, for example, that nasopharyngeal cancer is not on the list of AIDS indicator illnesses despite the fact that it is a common HIV-related cancer in Botswana. Patients who are diagnosed with this cancer are not automatically put on ARVs, though the oncologist would like them to be, unless their CD4 count is below the national threshold for initiating HAART (highly active antiretroviral therapy). I take the concept of local biology from Lock, *Encounters with Aging*.

17 Aronowitz, "Cancer Survivorship and the Entangled Experience of Disease and Risk."

18 The hood is a special table with a protective shield over it and built-in heavy rubber gloves used for mixing the (very toxic) drugs.

19 Mol, *The Body Multiple*, 64.

20 Livingston, *Debility and the Moral Imagination in Botswana*; Klaits, *Death in a Church of Life*.

21 I don't mean to imply that a clean break is made in the move from diagnosis to treatment. Treatment often necessitates or includes a number of diagnostic or monitoring procedures, and treatment itself is diagnostic. And in any case patients are not always clear which practices are meant to be purely diagnostic.

22 This is, of course, not unique to Africa. Stacy Pigg has written a great deal about this, showing how, for example, a seemingly universal domain of experience and practice like sex lacks a corresponding unitary signifier in Nepal. Thus AIDS peer-education programs founder or must unwittingly create entirely new objects through processes of language translation. See Pigg, "Globalizing the Facts of Life."

23 The day after a discussion of these "soldiers," I wrote in my field notes, "This is not the only reason I think of Susan Sontag here daily." See also Martin, *Flexible Bodies*.

24 Cohen, *A Body Worth Defending*.

25 Dr. P was, of course, quite concerned about iatrogenic wounds from chemo infiltration, and he took various precautions to prevent them. Tubes of steroids and maxolon (a mild anti-emetic) were always pushed first, to minimize extravasation if the cannula weren't properly situated in the vein. Often, extravasation wounds were caused by medical officers who lacked Dr. P's considerable skill in placing cannulas and who, moreover, were sometimes intensely ex-

hausted from having taken the night shift in the medical ward and thus arriving in oncology as part of a twenty-four-hour shift.

INTERLUDE ⚘ AMPUTATION DAY

1 I offer here an example of a piece of ethnography without a great deal of theoretical apparatus or analytic architecture, which is why it is titled as an interlude, rather than as a chapter. This is a moment which is not as thematically or analytically emplotted as the rest of the book, so that the reader can experience the forcefulness and complexity of the clinical space as a site of human drama. My intention is to present a piece of writing that by its very tone asks the reader to pause for a moment, to feel, to grapple with the pressures, the high stakes, the passions, tensions, crises, and the difficult choices of this place, the dystopia of redemption through cutting. As such, I hope it gives those who will read the book in the context of developing a better understanding of ethnography a clear and straightforward example of ethnography as a method of research conjoined to a mode of writing. For medical students, doctors, nurses, and patients, it also presents a moment in which they can see the pressures of the clinical from the outside in and contemplate or debate the complexities of clinical ethics, the narrowness of the clinical space in relation to the totality of the patient's life.

2 Nguyen, *The Republic of Therapy*.

3 Vaughan, *Curing Their Ills*.

FOUR ⚘ THE MORAL INTIMACIES OF CARE

1 Botswana, of course, is neither without faults, nor without political detractors. My point is not to evaluate its political fault lines, but rather to examine its processes of health-making. On political critique, see, for example, Werber, "Challenging Minorities, Differences, and Tribal Citizenship in Botswana." On botho, see Livingston, "Disgust, Bodily Aesthetics, and the Ethic of Being Human in Botswana."

2 See, for example, President Festus Mogae's State of the Nation Address in 2001, when he declared, "HIV/AIDS is the most serious challenge facing our nation, and a threat to our continued existence as a people." Mogae, "State of the Nation Address, 2001."

3 Vaughan, *Story of an African Famine*.

4 In this framing of harming and healing, and in my desire to see nurses as intellectuals (compare with Gramsci), I am following the lead of Steve Feierman. See Feierman, *The Shamba Kingdom*; Feierman, *Peasant Intellectuals*; and Feierman, "Struggles for Control."

5 See Klaits, *Death in a Church of Life*. In "Islam, Fatalism, and Medical Intervention," Sherine Hamdy describes a situation in Egypt where terminally ill dialysis patients draw on religious tenets to cultivate fortitude and to make meaning out of suffering and bodily demise. She argues that such efforts should be read

as strength and discipline (as patients themselves understand it), not as passivity or fatalism. Similar dynamics hold in PMH oncology.

6 In *A Colonial Lexicon of Birth Ritual, Medicalization, and Mobility in the Congo*, Nancy Hunt establishes African nurses as key "middle figures" in social health. See also Whyte, Whyte, and Kyaddondo, "Health Workers Entangled."

7 Kleinman, "Caregiving"; Tronto, *Moral Boundaries*; Mol, *The Logic of Care*; Garcia, *The Pastoral Clinic*.

8 This is also the case in South Africa, and perhaps the broader region. In South Africa, as Rachel Jewkes, Naeemah Abrahams, and Zodumo Mvo describe in "Why Do Nurses Abuse Patients?," patients accessing midwifery services face humiliation, neglect, and even abuse. Complaints about nursing in Botswana rarely, if ever, rise to this level. While people may complain that patients are neglected or that nurses are rude and intimidating, abuse does not seem to be at issue. In further contrast to the midwifery services Jewkes, Abrahams, and Mvo researched, oncology is a unique location, where nurses get to know many of their patients over time, and where patients are recognized to be quite ill. This is not to say that there is no complaint in oncology, or that complaints are never justified.

9 See, for example, Chaguturu and Vallabhaneni, "Aiding and Abetting"; and the special issue on global nurse migration in *Policy, Politics and Nursing Practice* 7.3, supplement (2006).

10 See, for example, the article "Princess Marina Wards Stink" in the government newspaper, the *Botswana Daily News* (accessed 28 February 2012), in which PMH nurses are both criticized and acknowledged as the backbone of the health system. Elise Carpenter has written an excellent study that demonstrates the creativity and commitment of nurses and their crucial role in developing and implementing ARV policy. Carpenter, "The Social Practice of HIV Drug Therapy in Botswana, 2002–2004," chap. 4.

11 "Closed Marina Hospital Wards to Be Reopened," accessed 9 February 2010.

12 "Botswana," accessed 5 February 2010. The nurses in PMH oncology are not "oncology nurses" per se, nor do they have the option to become so trained. Nurses in PMH are rotated every two years to new wards and duties, though some are able to remain in a ward through two rotations. They may have been a surgical scrub nurse in their last rotation, or headed to radiology or to labor and delivery on their next rotation. During most of my time at PMH, only Mma M, the ward matron, had specialist training in oncology, though in May 2009 she was joined by Rra T, who had just come from oncology training in South Africa. Nurses in Botswana receive little education about cancer during their training, so they enter the oncology ward having to learn the theoretical and practical knowledge on the fly. The difficulty of acquiring specialized skills contributes to Batswana nurses' complaints about compensation. Without the ability to specialize, it becomes difficult to find a pathway both for salary advancement and for developing the kind of expertise and personal advancement that brings satisfaction to professionals.

13 In this way hospital nursing is similar to the nursing care provided by female relatives in the home, which is also loaded with similar expectations and moral critique. See Livingston, *Debility and the Moral Imagination in Botswana*. Fred Klaits writes eloquently on the importance of sentiment to care in Botswana, in *Death in a Church of Life*.

14 Again, I have changed the names and some of the distinguishing details of various people here in an attempt to protect their anonymity. I am not describing an actual gynecology nurse!

15 One of the best in-depth discussions of nursing care issues is Benner and Wrubel, *The Primacy of Caring*. And surely the best contemporary ethnography is Theresa Brown, *Critical Care*.

16 Recent research indicates high levels of depression among people living with HIV. Lawler et al., "Depression among HIV-Positive Individuals in Botswana."

17 As I described in chapter 2, the plight of Zimbabwean patients, so in need of care, which is not extended to them free of charge, reinforces the meanings of citizenship in Botswana as a set of services and opportunities facilitated by moral governance. Expectations of medical care as intrinsic to citizenship in Botswana contrast with the model of urgent and uncertain biological citizenship Adriana Petryna describes for Ukrainians, in *Life Exposed*. By contrast, see also, Turshen, *Privatizing Health Services in Africa*; Nguyen, "Government by Exception." But this does mean that nurses are state actors, and as such they wield tremendous power in brokering the benefits of public medical care.

18 Ferguson, *Expectations of Modernity*.

19 There are certainly those who argue that the government should spend more on this or that project, but not that the nation should live beyond its means. In contrast to the government, many individuals live with serious debt. See Livingston, "Suicide, Risk, and Investment at the Heart of the African Miracle."

20 See, for example, Durham, "Soliciting Gifts and Negotiating Agency."

21 Of course, nurses worldwide have serious complaints about compensation, which drive some abroad in search of better remuneration, as well as out of the profession entirely. Though pay scales are higher in Botswana than in neighboring countries, nurses find it hard to fulfill their responsibilities and desires on their salaries. See Thupayagale-Tshweneagae, "Migration of Nurses."

22 This is comparable to the situation of rural Kenyan health assistants described by Patricia Kingori, in "What Constitutes a 'Good' Public Health Researcher in the Conduct of Fieldwork in Resource-Constrained Settings."

23 I am not claiming this to be the case in all cancer wards—see, by contrast, the excellent patient-centered ethnography by the anthropologist Benson A. Mulemi, "Coping with Cancer and Adversity."

24 The weekday morning shift is the best staffed. Depending on overall staffing levels, the afternoon/evening shift might have as few as two nurses, and the night shift is sometimes a solo endeavor.

25 I take the phrase "identified life" from King, "Fame and Fortune."

26 See Makoae, "The Phenomenology of Bodily Care."

27 When Dumisane first came to oncology, the previous month, and took off his hat, Dr. P noticed that he had a hole in his skull, which was not noted in his medical cards. With a flashlight, we could see straight into the dural matter. Dr. P and Dr. A were absolutely amazed that someone could be walking around with such a hole, and they brought the patient to Accident and Emergency, where seemingly every doctor in the hospital took a turn looking into the hole.

28 Livingston, *Debility and the Moral Imagination.*

29 Klaits, *Death in a Church of Life*; Werbner, *Holy Hustlers, Schism, and Prophecy.*

30 I discuss these feelings and their relationship to citizenship and Tswana moral sentiment in depth elsewhere. See Livingston, "Disgust, Bodily Aesthetics, and the Ethic of Being Human in Botswana." Disgust is a complicated and morally laden emotion. For further discussion, see Nussbaum, *Hiding from Humanity*; and Miller, *The Anatomy of Disgust.*

31 Janzen, *Quest for Therapy in Lower Zaire.*

32 I take this term from Robert Murphy, *The Body Silent.*

33 Jewkes, Abrahams, and Mvo, "Why Do Nurses Abuse Patients?" In Bangladesh, nurses are also potentially tainted by their bodily care for lower-class patients. Hadley et al., "Why Bangladeshi Nurses Avoid 'Nursing.'"

34 Of course what had happened was that the patient's friend had run to his mother's home with the news of his condition and mood. She had put her things together as the family pooled funds for her trip (fortunately it was mid-month, so there was still cash on hand), and she had departed then and there hurrying toward her son.

FIVE ◊ PAIN AND LAUGHTER

1 Human Rights Watch, *Unbearable Pain*; Human Rights Watch, *Needless Pain*; Krakauer, "Just Palliative Care."

2 Because of the lack of screening capacities, a majority of Botswana's cancer patients are diagnosed after their disease is already advanced. Such cancers are widely recognized to cause moderate to severe pain in the vast majority of patients. See Cleland, Nakamura, Mendoza, Edwards, Douglas, and Serlin, "Dimensions of the Impact of Cancer Pain in a Four Country Sample"; Daut and Cleland, "The Prevalence and Severity of Pain in Cancer"; Portenoy and Lesage, "Management of Cancer Pain"; Foley, "Pain Syndromes in Patients with Cancer."

3 The functioning and structure of the broader health system also matters here. The presence of drugs themselves and the universal healthcare system that provides them free to patients are critical to the ethic of palliation. It is instructive to compare this ethic of palliation with the situation described in Kenya's central referral hospital by the anthropologist B. A. Mulemi in "Coping with Cancer and Adversity."

4 Scarry, *The Body in Pain.*

5 Interviews with Tshenolo Thebe and Difelo Botsang, in Kumakwane, 7 Decem-

ber 2006; Mmatli Rannokgwane, in Thamaga, 10 December 2006; Mma Mant-shadi, Ikgopoleng Keoreme, Ketlantshang Piet, and Omphemetse Piet, in Kumakwane, 9 December 2006; Modise Thebe, in Kumakwane, 15 December 2006; Modisaetsile Thapelo, in Kumakwane, 15 December 2006. Tapes and transcripts of interviews are in the author's possession.

6 Pain medicines, however, do have a thingy-ness. Patients are clear that some medicines are "painkillers," separating pain from pathology. This dynamic of separation and attendant individuation around pain (in dentistry) has been beautifully articulated by the historian Paul Landau in relation to early-twentieth-century mission practice, in "Explaining Surgical Evangelism in Colonial Southern Africa."

7 Asad, *Formations of the Secular*, 85. See also Das, "Language and the Body."

8 Pethidine is a strong synthetic opioid. American readers may be familiar with its brand name, Demerol.

9 Later, there was debate as to why the bone had not been disarticulated, with the surgeons arguing that M himself had requested to keep as much of his thigh as possible, balking at the loss of the femur. My point is not to showcase surgical failure, however, for I am not qualified to judge who, if anyone, was at fault in this case of amputation gone wrong.

10 On pain being in doubt, see Scarry, *The Body in Pain*.

11 Pain assessment has been part of nursing training in Botswana since the mid-1970s, but it is not integral to daily practice in the hospitals and clinics. See Irene Manyere, "The Uses of the Pain Assessment Tools by Nurses in Botswana in Assessing and Managing Pain," 3.

12 Donald McNeil, "Drugs Banned, World's Poor Suffer in Pain," *New York Times*, 10 September 2007; Logie and Leng, "Africans Die in Pain because of Fears of Opiate Addiction"; World Health Organization, *A Community Health Approach to Palliative Care for* HIV/AIDS *and Cancer Patients*. For better or for worse, palliative care has become an umbrella in African healthcare, where everything from the writing of wills to the provision of soap and nutritional education is promoted. In such a configuration, attention to bodily pain may be compromised by the vast array of problems in need of attention. At one ministry of health palliative-care workshop I attended, where we were charged with reviewing the new palliative-care guidelines for different levels of the health system, we spent much more time discussing these other (admittedly important) issues than discussing pain.

13 See, for example, Mosweunyane, "The Knowledge of Nurses working in Botswana Health Care Settings in Regard to Pain Control"; Moyo, "The Extent to which Nurses Meet Clients' Needs for Pain Management within the First 48 Hours Post C-Section."

14 World Health Organization, *A Community Health Approach to Palliative Care for* HIV/AIDS *and Cancer Patients*, 25.

15 Murray, Grant, Grant, and Kendall, "Dying from Cancer in Developed and Developing Countries," 368.

16 International Narcotics Control Board, *Report of the International Narcotics Control Board for 2004*, cited in University of Wisconsin Pain and Policy Studies Group, *Availability of Morphine and Pethidine in the World and Africa*, 4.

17 In *Availability of Morphine and Pethidine in the World and Africa*, the University of Wisconsin Pain and Policy Studies Group, a WHO center, explains the metric of morphine equivalence: "Historically, the WHO has considered a country's annual consumption of morphine to be an indicator of the extent that opioids are used to treat severe cancer pain and an index to evaluate improvements in pain management. However, over the past 20 years additional opioid analgesic medications and formulations, such as the fentanyl patch, hydromorphone, and sustained-release oxycodone, have been introduced in global and national markets and should be considered when studying opioid consumption in a country, region, and globally. Using the INCB [International Narcotics Control Board] data it receives annually, and applying conversion factors from the WHO Collaborating Center for Drugs Statistics Methodology, PPSG [Pain and Policy Study Group] developed a Morphine Equivalence (ME) metric, adjusted for population, for 6 principal opioids used to treat moderate to severe pain."

18 University of Wisconsin Pain and Policy Studies Group, *Availability of Morphine and Pethidine in the World and Africa*, table 1. These statistics need to be taken with a grain of salt. Some necessary figures appear to be missing, and there are some dramatic and unexplained spikes. Distribution through Central Medical Stores, Botswana's national centralized pharmaceutical-procurement system, has been problematic, as it scales up the quantity and array of drugs available in the face of changing epidemiological norms, the AIDS epidemic in particular, and as attempts to localize purchasing and distribution continue. It is not my aim to pin down exact figures, but rather to make the general point, which can be supported by the statistics, that despite large numbers of desperately sick people, strong painkillers are not widely used in Botswana. I am also not arguing that more is always better; overmedication and drug addiction are real problems that should not be overlooked, and some of these dynamics are no doubt hidden within the large American aggregate figure.

19 Koshy et al., "Cancer Pain Management in Developing Countries."

20 Mosweunyane, "The Knowledge of Nurses Working in Botswana Health Care Settings in Regard to Pain Control," 26.

21 Yet, at times, I also found myself—an ethnographer with no medical training—being the one to suggest or request that a patient receive pethidine before wound cleaning or a prescription for morphine tablets for use at home. This, I think, was the result of the pressures of work, in this setting where the oncologist worked seven days a week, and where nurses were not only occupied in the ward and clinic, but also often with caring for their own patients at home. The attitude of nurses on the oncology ward was quite different from those of nurses in the medical and surgical wards, where some doctors (mainly European or American expatriates) and one Motswana nursing professor complained about the reluctance of nurses to administer strong pain relief;

yet when I accompanied staff on their rounds, I found that the same doctors often did not explicitly ask patients about pain. Nurses in Botswana are shifted among posts every two years, so the differences cannot be accounted for by assuming that oncology nurses had special training in oncology. Instead, I attribute the marked difference in approaches to pain relief among hospital domains mainly to the strong personality of the oncologist, and to the oncology training and ethos of compassion of the nursing matron in charge of the cancer ward.

22　See, for example, Kennedy, "Chronic Sore Throat."

23　Lock, *Encounters with Aging*, 39.

24　Lock, *Encounters with Aging*; Lock and Nguyen, *An Anthropology of Biomedicine*.

25　I had seen Dr. P do bone marrow biopsies already, and I understood the purpose. But after my conversation with O, I wanted to double-check my understanding of the procedure, so I got on the Internet. The WebMD and the Mayo Clinic websites both described the procedure to their presumably middle-class (Internet-accessing) American patients, who learn they may receive a sedative, and who would presumably be provided with a hospital gown to wear during the procedure. The contrast between the description provided online and what I witnessed is instructive. See "Bone Marrow Aspiration and Biopsy," and "Bone Marrow Biopsy and Aspiration," both accessed 28 February 2012.

26　Mma Mantshadi, Ikgopoleng Keoreme, Ketlantshang Piet, and Omphemetse Piet, interview by author, Kumakwane, 9 December 2006; Naomi Seboni, personal communication, December 2006.

27　Livingstone, *Missionary Travels and Researches in South Africa*, 145.

28　Haltunnen, "Humanitarianism and the Pornography of Pain in Anglo-American Culture"; Foucault, *Discipline and Punish*.

29　Pernick, *A Calculus of Suffering*, 104.

30　Ibid.

31　Ibid.

32　See also Fabian, *Out of Our Minds*.

33　Mack, *Heart Religion in the Early Enlightenment*.

34　Thomson, "Journey of the Society's East African Expedition," 723.

35　Phillips, "The Lower Congo," 217.

36　Roche, *On Trek in the Transvaal*, 177–78.

37　Wood, *The Uncivilized Races of Men in All Countries of the World*, 240.

38　Ibid., 230.

39　Ibid., 531. There are numerous other references to pain in this volume, which synthesizes (or perhaps plagiarizes is a more accurate term) the writings of countless travelers.

40　Price, *Journals Written in Bechuanaland*, 82, entry Mashuwe, 21 November 1862.

41　Stoneham, "Origin of Cruelty," 248.

42　Dirks, "The Policing of Tradition"; Ko, *Cinderella's Sisters*; Thomas, *The Politics of the Womb: Women, Reproduction, and the State in Kenya*; Pederson, "National Bodies, Unspeakable Acts."

43 See, for example, Smuts, "Native Policy in Africa," 250; Sloley, "The African Native Labour Contingent and the Welfare Committee," 206.

44 Woodworth, "Racial Differences in Mental Traits," 177.

45 Loram, *The Education of the South African Native*, 194–95. See also Mumford and Smith, "Racial Comparisons and Intelligence Testing." Mumford and Smith also refer to Woodworth's research at the World's Fair in St. Louis in 1904, which tested about three hundred people of different non-European groups—"American Indians, Eskimaux, Patagonians . . . Africans, and a few Pygmies from the Congo"—for differences in pain (49).

46 Pernick, *A Calculus of Suffering*, 155.

47 Fleure, "Racial Evolution and Archaeology," 210.

48 Seligman, "Anthropological Perspective and Psychological Theory."

49 Kuper, "The Colonial Situation in Southern Africa," 160.

50 Zoborowski, *People in Pain*, chap. 1.

51 Ibid.

52 See, for example, Vaughan, *Curing Their Ills*; Jackson, *Surfacing Up*; and Sadowsky, *Imperial Bedlam*.

53 See, for example, Kennedy, "Chronic Sore Throat."

54 Batswana are not alone in this sensibility—in fact, I have found it quite instructive to read the letter of the early-nineteenth-century British author Fanny Burney in which she recounts her mastectomy, which was performed in her home in Paris in 1812. I am grateful to Mary Fissell for conversation and insight on these matters.

55 The specifics of *bogwera* (male initiation) and *bojale* (female initiation) varied between *morafe* (sub-ethnic chiefdom) and are difficult to uncover since all initiates, male and female, took vows to preserve the secrecy of the initiation rites. Nonetheless, the missionaries Rev. J. Tom Brown and Rev. W. C. Willoughby and the anthropologist Isaac Schapera were able to gather some information from initiated informants about bogwera practices. The following is based on their accounts. Willoughby, "Notes on the Initiation Ceremonies of the Becwana"; Rev. J. Tom Brown, "Circumcision Rites of the Becwana Tribes"; Schapera, *Bogwera*. For a more thorough discussion of bojale specifically, see Comaroff, *Body of Power, Spirit of Resistance*, 114–18.

56 Schapera, *Bogwera*.

57 Landau, "Explaining Surgical Evangelism in Colonial Southern Africa."

58 Mma Mantshadi, Ikgopoleng Keoreme, Ketlantshang Piet, and Omphemetse Piet, interview by author, Kumakwane, 16 November 2006; Merriweather, *Desert Doctor*; Anderson and Staugart, *Traditional Midwives*.

59 Anderson and Staugart, *Traditional Midwives*, 130.

60 Ibid. This resonates with what I witnessed during births I attended on the Ob-Gyn night shift in PMH in 2007.

61 Haram, "A Child Is Born"; and Anderson and Staugart, "Modern Maternity Care."

62 Elderly men slipping in and out of consciousness also might moan or cry out—but I associate this with the loss of consciousness.

63 Livingston, "Suicide, Risk, and Investment in the Heart of the African Miracle."

64 Pain and childbirth is a highly significant topic, but a more thorough exposition would need its own study.

65 Landau, "Explaining Surgical Evangelism in Colonial Southern Africa."

66 See also Brown, *Critical Care.*

67 For Botswana, see Werbner, *Holy Hustlers, Schism, and Prophecy*; Klaits, *Death in a Church of Life.* Writing about Tanzania, in *Bodies, Politics, and African Healing*, Stacey Langwick refers to these experiences as part of the "intimate becoming" of healers.

68 Interviews with Tshenolo Thebe and Difelo Botsang, in Kumakwane, 7 December 2006; Mmatli Rannokgwane, in Thamaga, 10 December 2006; Mma Mantshadi, Ikgopoleng Keoreme, Ketlantshang Piet, and Omphemetse Piet, in Kumakwane, 9 December 2006; Modise Thebe, in Kumakwane, 15 December 2006; Modisaetsile Thapelo, in Kumakwane, 15 December 2006. All interview recordings in author's possession.

SIX ◊ DURING CANCER, BEFORE DEATH

1 Aronowitz, *Unnatural History*; Gina Kolata, "Advances Elusive in Drive to Cure Cancer," *New York Times*, 23 April 2009; Natasha Singer, "In Push for Cancer Screening, Limited Benefits," *New York Times*, 16 July 2009.

2 I am especially grateful to Tim Burke for his thoughts on this.

3 Hamdy, "When the State and Your Kidneys Fail"; Kaufman, *And a Time to Die*; Larkin, *Signal and Noise.*

4 Kaufman, *And a Time to Die*; Lock, *Twice Dead.*

5 Mol, *The Logic of Care.*

6 Triage, as Vinh-Kim Nguyen explains, is a concept that "was developed on the battlefield, as a way to use scarce treatment resources in the most rational way: those most likely to live are prioritized to receive care, while those whose prognosis is poor are left to die" (*The Republic of Therapy*, 100). Nguyen then extends this logic in his analysis of the global and local politics governing the distribution of therapies for HIV/AIDS. By contrast, in *And a Time to Die*, Sharon Kaufman, who worked in American community hospitals (and who does not use the term *triage*), demonstrates how end-of-life care is triaged via a sense of urgency and action generated by certain biological processes (cardiac arrest and respiratory arrest), combined with bureaucracies that dictate which services are compensated and which not. To some extent, the situation in PMH oncology evidences a mix of these two possibilities. Here I examine a triage situation in the ward marked in part by a tension between how scarce resources are distributed in ways that both prioritize a sense of urgency over the care meant to stabilize the critically ill, and also prioritize care for those with better prognoses.

7 No doubt for others the dynamic works in reverse, with relatives of dying

patients avoiding PMH based on past experience. This avoidance of the hospital as a house of death is a long-standing trope in discussions of African health-seeking strategies. Such avoidance is a reasonable and pragmatic response to the conditions of many African hospitals and the fees they now charge (Botswana being an exception in this regard). What is significant here is the extent to which this is *not* the case in PMH oncology.

8 Didion, *The Year of Magical Thinking.*

9 See also Levy, "Communicating with the Cancer Patient in Zimbabwe."

10 Harris, Shao, and Sugarman, "Disclosure of Cancer Diagnosis and Prognosis in Northern Tanzania."

11 These changes are not as radical, however, as we are often led to believe. As the clinician-scholar Robert Aronowitz notes, "Looking at the history of doctor-patient interactions one sees more continuities than discontinuities" (*Unnatural History*, 17). He goes on to suggest that a historical awareness of these "currents . . . might make us more skeptical about the idealized patient-consumer role and more aware of the complexity and tragedy of action when hope and honesty are in conflict" (ibid., 17).

12 These dynamics have been critiqued to great effect by medical anthropologists and historians. See, for example, Briggs and Mantini-Briggs, *Stories in the Time of Cholera*; Packard, *White Plague, Black Labor*; Vaughn, *Curing Their Ills.*

13 Klaits, *Death in a Church of Life.*

14 Gordon and Paci, "Disclosure Practices and Cultural Narratives."

15 Livingston, *Debility and the Moral Imagination in Botswana.*

16 Butow, Hagerty, Tattersall, and Stockler, "Foretelling"; Gordon and Paci, "Disclosure Practices and Cultural Narratives."

17 Rieff, *Swimming in a Sea of Death.*

18 Kaufman, *And a Time to Die.*

19 Christakis, *Death Foretold*; Groopman, *How Doctors Think.*

20 Harris, Shao, and Sugarman, "Disclosure of Cancer Diagnosis and Prognosis in Northern Tanzania." See also Solanke, "Communication with the Cancer Patient in Nigeria."

21 Lavi, *The Modern Art of Dying*, 54.

22 Good, Good, Schaffer, and Lind, "American Oncology and the Discourse of Hope"; Ehrenreich, "Pathologies of Hope."

23 Jain, "Living in Prognosis"; Aronowitz, *Unnatural History*; Proctor, *Cancer Wars.*

24 Jain, "Cancer Butch."

25 Miyakazi, *The Method of Hope.*

26 Livingston, "AIDS as Chronic Illness."

EPILOGUE ⟱ CHANGING WARDS,
FURTHER IMPROVISATIONS

1 Ferguson, *Expectations of Modernity*.
2 Turshen, *Privatizing Health Services in Africa*.
3 Mutizwa-Mangiza, *Doctors and the State*; Gaidzanwa, "Voting with Their Feet."
4 Knapp, "World Report."
5 Ndlovu, "Mpilo Doctors Revolt over 'Appalling Work Conditions,'" accessed 7 April 2011; "Zimbabwe: Recession Hits Renal Patients," accessed 7 April 2011; Adams, "Zimbabwe."
6 The patient in question had HIV and was on antiretrovirals. A senior internist explained to me that given the emphasis on providing HIV drugs in many global programs, from Médicins Sans Frontières to the Global Fund, antiretrovirals were currently available in Bulawayo, but not so the many drugs and technologies needed to manage the complications of the disease.
7 "Mpilo General Surgical Centre Shut Down," accessed 8 April 2011.

Abdullahi, Najad. "'Toxic Waste' behind Somali Piracy." *Al Jazeera*, 11 October 2008, http://english.aljazeera.net.

Adams, Kate. "Zimbabwe: An Eyewitness Account." *British Medical Journal* 336 (12 January 2008): 98.

Anderson, Sandra, and Frants Staugart. "Modern Maternity Care: Two Case Studies." *Traditional Midwives: Traditional Medicine in Botswana*, Sandra Anderson and Frants Staugart, 53–60. Gaborone: Ipelegeng Publishers, 1986.

———. *Traditional Midwives: Traditional Medicine in Botswana*. Gaborone: Ipelegeng Publishers, 1986.

Aronowitz, Robert. "Cancer Survivorship and the Entangled Experience of Disease and Risk." Unpublished manuscript.

———. "The Converged Experience of Risk and Disease." *Milbank Quarterly* 87.2 (June 2009): 417–42.

———. *Unnatural History: Breast Cancer and American Society*. New York: Cambridge University Press, 2007.

Asad, Talal. *Formations of the Secular: Christianity, Islam, Modernity*. Palo Alto: Stanford University Press, 2003.

Benner, Patricia, and Judith Wrubel. *The Primacy of Caring: Stress and Coping in Health and Illness*. Reading, Mass.: Addison Wesley Longman, 1989.

Biehl, João. "The Activist State: Global Pharmaceuticals, AIDS, and Citizenship in Brazil." *Social Text* 22.3 (2004): 105–32.

———. "Pharmaceuticalization: AIDS Treatment and Global Health Politics." *Anthropological Quarterly* 80.4 (2007): 1083–126.

———. *Vita: Life in a Zone of Social Abandonment*. Berkeley: University of California Press, 2005.

"Bone Marrow Aspiration and Biopsy." WebMD, http://www.webmd.com/.

"Bone Marrow Biopsy and Aspiration." MayoClinic, http://www.mayoclinic.com/.

Bosk, Charles. *Forgive and Remember: Managing Medical Failure*. Chicago: University of Chicago Press, 2003.

"Botswana: Bleak Outlook for Future AIDS Funding." IRIN Plus News: Global HIV/AIDS News and Analysis 2009, http://www.irinnews.org.

"Botswana: Main Referral Hospital Facing Crisis." IRIN Humanitarian News and Analysis, 22 September 2004, http://www.irinnews.org.

Boyle, P., et al. "Editorial: Need for Global Action for Cancer Control." *Annals of Oncology* 19 (2008): 1519–21.

Boyle, Peter, and Bernard Levin, eds. *World Cancer Report 2008*. Lyon: World Health Organization / International Agency for Research on Cancer, 2008.

Brada, Betsey. "Botswana as a Living Experiment." PhD diss., Department of Anthropology, University of Chicago, 2011.

———. "'Not *Here*': Making the Spaces and Subjects of 'Global Health' in Botswana." *Culture, Medicine and Psychiatry* 35 (2011): 285–312.

Brandt, Allan. *The Cigarette Century: The Rise, Fall, and Deadly Persistence of the Product That Defined America*. New York: Basic Books, 2007.

Braun, Lundy. "Structuring Silence: Asbestos and Biomedical Research in Britain and South Africa." *Race and Class* 50.1 (2008): 59–78.

Braun, Lundy, and Sophia Kisting. "Asbestos-Related Disease in South Africa: The Social Production of an Invisible Epidemic." *American Journal of Public Health* 96.8 (August 2006): 1386–96.

Braun, Lundy, and Ling Phoun. "HPV Vaccination Campaigns: Masking Uncertainty, Erasing Complexity." *The HPV Vaccine and Sexual Risk: Citizens and States at the Crossroads of Cancer Prevention*, ed. Keith Wailoo, Julie Livingston, Stephen Epstein, and Robert Aronowitz, 39–60. Baltimore: Johns Hopkins University Press, 2010.

Briggs, Charles, and Clara Mantini-Briggs. *Stories in the Time of Cholera: Racial Profiling during a Medical Nightmare*. Berkeley: University of California Press, 2004.

Brown, Rev. J. Tom. "Circumcision Rites of the Becwana Tribes." *Journal of the Royal Anthropological Institute of Great Britain and Ireland* 51 (1922): 419–27.

Brown, Theresa. *Critical Care: A New Nurse Faces Life, Death, and Everything In Between*. New York: HarperOne, 2010.

Burkitt, D. P., and S. K. Kyalwazi. "Spontaneous Remission of African Lymphoma." *British Journal of Cancer* 21.1 (1967): 14–16.

Bussmann, H., et al. "Five-Year Outcomes of Initial Patients Treated in Botswana's National Antiretroviral Treatment Program." *AIDS* 22 (2008): 2303–11.

Butow, Phyllis, Rebecca Hagerty, Martin Tattersall, and Martin Stockler. "Foretelling: Communicating the Prognosis." *Prognosis in Advanced Cancer*, ed. Paul Glare and Nicholas Christakis, 33–53. New York: Oxford University Press, 2008.

Caldwell, J., P. Caldwell, and P. Quiggin. "The Social Context of AIDS in Sub-Saharan Africa." *Population and Development Review* 15.2 (1989): 185–234.

Carpenter, Elise. "The Social Practice of HIV Drug Therapy in Botswana, 2002–

2004: Experts, Bureaucrats, and Healthcare Providers." PhD diss., History and Sociology of Science, University of Pennsylvania, 2008.

Central Intelligence Agency. *The World Fact Book, 2010*, https://www.cia.gov.

Chaguturu, Sreekanth, and Snigdha Vallabhaneni. "Aiding and Abetting: Nursing Crises at Home and Abroad." *New England Journal of Medicine* 353.17 (27 October 2005): 1761–63.

Christakis, Nicholas. *Death Foretold: Prophesy and Progress in Medical Care*. Chicago: University of Chicago Press, 2001.

Clapp, Jennifer. *Toxic Exports: The Transfer of Hazardous Wastes from Rich to Poor Countries*. Ithaca: Cornell University Press, 2001.

Cleland, C. S., Y. Nakamura, T. R. Mendoza, K. R. Edwards, J. Douglas, and R. C. Serlin. "Dimensions of the Impact of Cancer Pain in a Four Country Sample: New Information from Multidimensional Scaling." *Pain* 67 (1996): 2–3, 267–73.

"Closed Marina Hospital Wards to Be Reopened." *Botswana Daily News*, 10 April 2001, http://www.dailynews.gov.

Cohen, Ed. *A Body Worth Defending: Immunity, Biopolitics, and the Apotheosis of the Modern Body*. Durham: Duke University Press, 2009.

Comaroff, Jean. *Body of Power, Spirit of Resistance: The Culture and History of a South African People*. Chicago: University of Chicago Press, 1985.

———. "The Diseased Heart of Africa: Medicine, Colonialism, and the Black Body." *Knowledge, Power, and Practice: The Anthropology of Medicine and Everyday Life*, ed. Shirley Lindenbaum and Margaret Lock, 305–29. Berkeley: University of California Press, 1993.

Creek, T. L., et al. "Successful Introduction of Routine Opt-Out HIV Testing in Antenatal Care in Botswana." *Journal of AIDS* 45 (2007): 102–7.

Culliton, Barbara J. "Cancer: Select Committee Calls Virus Program a Closed Shop." *Science* 182.4117 (14 December 1973): 1110–12.

Dahl, Bianca. "Left Behind? Orphaned Children and the Politics of Kinship, Culture, and Caregiving during Botswana's AIDS Crisis." PhD diss., University of Chicago, 2009.

Das, Veena. "Language and the Body: Transactions in the Construction of Pain." *Social Suffering*, ed. Arthur Kleinman, Veena Das, and Margaret Lock, 67–92. Berkeley: University of California Press, 1997.

Daut, R. L., and C. S. Cleland. "The Prevalence and Severity of Pain in Cancer." *Cancer* 50 (1982): 1913–18.

Denny, Lynette, Michael Quinn, and R. Sankaranarayanan. "Screening for Cervical Cancer in Developing Countries." *Vaccine* 24.S3 (2006): 71–77.

Didion, Joan. *The Year of Magical Thinking*. New York: Knopf, 2005.

Dirks, Nicholas. "The Policing of Tradition: Colonialism and Anthropology in Southern India." *Comparative Studies in Society and History* 39.1 (1997): 182–212.

Dow, Unity, and Max Essex. *Saturday Is for Funerals*. Cambridge: Harvard University Press, 2010.

Durham, Deborah. "Soliciting Gifts and Negotiating Agency: The Spirit of Asking in Botswana." *Journal of the Royal Anthropological Institute* 1 (1995): 111–28.

Durham, Deborah, and Frederick Klaits. "Funerals and the Public Space of Sentiment in Botswana." *Journal of Southern African Studies* 28.4 (December 2002): 777–95.

Durosinmi-Etti, F. A., M. Nofal, and M. M. Mahfouz. "Radiotherapy in Africa: Current Needs and Prospects." *IAEA Bulletin* 4 (1991): 24, 25.

Ecks, Stefan. "Global Pharmaceutical Markets and Corporate Citizenship: The Case of Novartis' Anti-cancer Drug Glivec." *Biosocieties* 3 (2008): 165–81.

Ehrenreich, Barbara. "Pathologies of Hope." *Harper's Magazine*, 1 February 2007.

Engels, E. A., et al. "Tuberculosis and Subsequent Risk of Lung Cancer in Xuanwei, China." *International Journal of Cancer* 124 (2009): 1183–87.

Fabian, Johannes. *Out of Our Minds: Reason and Madness in the Exploration of Central Africa*. Berkeley: University of California Press, 2000.

———. *Time and the Other: How Anthropology Makes Its Object*. New York: Columbia University Press, 1983.

Farmer, Paul, et al. "Expansion of Cancer Care and Control in Countries of Low and Middle Income: A Call to Action." *The Lancet* 6736.10 (2010): 1186–93.

Fassin, Didier. *When Bodies Remember: Experiences and Politics of AIDS in South Africa*. Berkeley: University of California Press, 2007.

Feierman, Steven. *Peasant Intellectuals: Anthropology and History in Tanzania*. Madison: University of Wisconsin Press, 1990.

———. *The Shamba Kingdom*. Madison: University of Wisconsin Press, 1974.

———. "Struggles for Control: The Social Roots of Health and Healing in Africa." *African Studies Review* 2.3 (1985): 73–147.

———. "When Physicians Meet: Local Medical Knowledge and Global Public Goods." *Evidence, Ethos, and Experiment: The Ethnography of Medical Research in Africa*, ed. Wenzel Geissler and Sassy Molyneaux, 171–96. New York: Berghahn, 2011.

Feigal, Ellen, and Jodi Black. "Cancer and AIDS: National Cancer Institute's Investment in Research." *Research Initiative/Treatment Action! Newsletter* (summer 2003): 26–29.

Feigal, Ellen, Alexandra Levine, and Robert Biggar, eds. *AIDS-Related Cancers and Their Treatment*. New York: Marcel Dekker, 2000.

Ferguson, James. *Expectations of Modernity: Myths and Meanings of Urban Life on the Zambian Copperbelt*. Berkeley: University of California Press, 1999.

Finkler, Kaja, Cynthia Hunter, and Rick Idema. "What Is Going On? Ethnography in Hospital Spaces." *Journal of Contemporary Ethnography* 37.2 (2008): 246–50.

Fleure, H. J. "Racial Evolution and Archaeology." *Journal of the Royal Anthropological Institute of Great Britain and Ireland* 67 (June 1937): 205–29.

Foley, K. M. "Pain Syndromes in Patients with Cancer." *Advances in Pain Research and Therapy*, ed. K. M. Foley, J. J. Bonica, and V. Ventafridda, 59–75. New York: Raven Press, 1979.

Foucault, Michel. *Discipline and Punish: The Birth of the Prison*. New York: Vintage, 1995.

Gaidzanwa, Rudo. *Voting with Their Feet: Migrant Zimbabwean Nurses and Doctors in the Era of Structural Adjustment.* Research Report no. 111. Uppsala: Nordiska Afrikainstitutet, 1999.

Garcia, Angela. *The Pastoral Clinic: Addiction and Dispossession along the Rio Grande.* Berkeley: University of California Press, 2010.

Geissler, Wenzel, and Ruth Prince. *The Land Is Dying: Contingency, Creativity, and Conflict in Western Kenya.* New York: Berghahn, 2010.

Gerrets, Rene. "Globalizing International Health: The Cultural Politics of 'Partnership' in Tanzanian Malaria Control." PhD diss., New York University, 2010.

Good, Mary-Jo DelVecchio. "The Biotechnical Embrace." *Culture, Medicine and Psychiatry* 25.4 (2001): 395–410.

Good, Mary-Jo DelVecchio, Byron Good, Cynthia Schaffer, and Stuart Lind. "American Oncology and the Discourse of Hope." *Culture, Medicine, and Psychiatry* 14.1 (1990): 59–79.

Gordon, Deborah, and Eugenio Paci. "Disclosure Practices and Cultural Narratives: Understanding Concealment and Silence around Cancer in Tuscany, Italy." *Social Science and Medicine* 44.10 (1997): 1433–52.

Groopman, Jerome. *How Doctors Think.* Boston: Houghton Mifflin, 2007.

Guindon, G. E. Emmanuel, and David Boscar. *Past, Current, and Future Trends in Tobacco Use.* International Bank for Reconstruction and Development / World Bank, 2003.

Hadley, Mary B., et al. "Why Bangladeshi Nurses Avoid 'Nursing': Social and Structural Factors on Hospital Wards in Bangladesh." *Social Science and Medicine* 64 (2007): 1166–77.

Haltunnen, Karen. "Humanitarianism and the Pornography of Pain in Anglo-American Culture." *American Historical Review* 100.2 (1995): 303–34.

Hamdy, Sherine. "Islam, Fatalism, and Medical Intervention: Lessons from Egypt on the Cultivation of Forbearance (Sabr) and Reliance on God." *Anthropological Quarterly* 82.1 (2009): 173–96.

———. "When the State and Your Kidneys Fail." *American Ethnologist* 35.4 (2008): 553–69.

Haram, Liv. "A Child Is Born: A Naturalistic Observation." *Traditional Midwives: Traditional Medicine in Botswana,* Sandra Anderson, and Frants Staugart, 129–34. Gaborone: Ipelegeng Publishers, 1986.

Harris, Julian, John Shao, and Jeremy Sugarman. "Disclosure of Cancer Diagnosis and Prognosis in Northern Tanzania." *Social Science and Medicine* 56 (2003): 905–13.

Haug, Charlotte J. "Human Papillomavirus Vaccination: Reasons for Caution." *New England Journal of Medicine* 359 (2008): 861–62.

Heald, Suzette. "It's Never as Easy as ABC: Understandings of AIDS in Botswana." *African Journal of AIDS Research* 1.1 (2002): 1–11.

———. "The Power of Sex: Some Reflections on the Caldwells' 'African Sexuality' Thesis." *Africa* 65 (1995): 489–505.

Hecht, Gabrielle. "Africa and the Nuclear World: Labor, Occupational Health, and the Transnational Production of Uranium." *Comparative Studies in Society and History* 51.4 (2009): 896–926.

———. *Being Nuclear: Africa and the Global Uranium Trade*. Cambridge: Massachusetts Institute of Technology Press, 2012.

———. "Hopes for the Radiated Body: Uranium Miners and Transnational Technopolitics in Namibia." *Journal of African History* 51 (2010): 213–34.

Higginson, John. "From Geographic Pathology to Environmental Carcinogenesis: A Historical Reminiscence." *Cancer Letters* 117 (1997): 133–42.

———. "The International Agency for Research on Cancer: A Brief Review of Its History, Mission, and Program." *Toxicological Sciences* 43 (1998): 79–85.

Human Rights Watch. *Needless Pain: Government Failure to Provide Palliative Care for Children in Kenya*. New York: Human Rights Watch, 2010.

———. *Unbearable Pain: India's Obligation to Ensure Palliative Care*. New York: Human Rights Watch, 2009.

Hunt, Nancy Rose. *A Colonial Lexicon of Birth Ritual, Medicalization, and Mobility in the Congo*. Durham: Duke University Press, 1999.

———. *A Nervous State: Violence, Remedies and Reverie in Colonial Congo*. Durham: Duke University Press, forthcoming.

Hunter, Mark. *Love in the Time of AIDS: Inequality, Gender, and Rights in South Africa*. Bloomington: Indiana University Press, 2010.

Iliffe, John. *East African Doctors: A History of the Modern Profession*. Cambridge: Cambridge University Press, 1998.

International Narcotics Control Board. *Report of the International Narcotics Control Board for 2004*. New York: United Nations, 2005.

Jackson, Lynette. *Surfacing Up: Psychiatry and Social Order in Colonial Zimbabwe*. Ithaca: Cornell University Press, 2005.

Jain, Sarah Lochlann. "Cancer Butch." *Cultural Anthropology* 22.4 (2007): 501–38.

———. "Living in Prognosis: Towards an Elegiac Politics." *Representations* 98 (spring 2007): 77–92.

———. "The Mortality Effect: Counting the Dead in the Cancer Trial." *Public Culture* 22.1 (2010): 89–117.

Janzen, John. *Quest for Therapy in Lower Zaire: Medical Pluralism in Lower Zaire*. Berkeley: University of California Press, 1982.

Jewkes, Rachel, Naeemah Abrahams, and Zodumo Mvo. "Why Do Nurses Abuse Patients? Reflections from South African Obstetric Services." *Social Science and Medicine* 47.11 (1998): 1781–95.

Johnson, R. H. "The Cases of Cancer Seen at a Botswana Hospital 1968-1972." *Central African Journal of Medicine* 21.12 (December 1975): 260–64.

Kalofonos, Ippolytos. "All I Eat Is ARVs: The Paradox of AIDS Treatment Interventions in Central Mozambique." *Medical Anthropology Quarterly* 24.3 (2010): 363–80.

Kark, S. L. "The Social Pathology of Syphilis in Africans." *South African Medical Journal* 23 (1949): 77–84.

Kaufman, Sharon. *And a Time to Die: How American Hospitals Shape the End of Life*. Chicago: University of Chicago Press, 2005.

Keirns, Carla. "Dying of a Treatable Disease." *Health Affairs* 25.6 (2009): 1807–13.

Kennedy, Dr. I. "Chronic Sore Throat: Antibiotics Down the Drain." *Botshelo: Journal of the Medical and Dental Association of Botswana* 11–12 (1–4): 28–31.

King, Nancy. "Fame and Fortune: The Simple Ethics of Organ Transplantation." *A Death Retold: Jesica Santillan, the Bungled Transplant, and Paradoxes of Medical Citizenship*, ed. Keith Wailoo, Julie Livingston, and Peter Guarnaccia, 349–60. Chapel Hill: University of North Carolina Press, 2006.

King, Nicholas B. "Security, Disease, Commerce: Ideologies of Postcolonial Global Health." *Social Studies of Science* 32.5–6 (2002): 763–89.

Kingori, Patricia. "What Constitutes a 'Good' Public Health Researcher in the Conduct of Fieldwork in Resource-Constrained Settings." Paper presented at the Publics of African Public Health Conference, Kilifi, Kenya, December 2009.

Klaits, Frederick. *Death in a Church of Life: Moral Passion in Botswana's Time of AIDS*. Berkeley: University of California Press, 2010.

Kleinman, Arthur. "Caregiving: The Odyssey of Becoming More Human." *The Lancet* 373 (24 January 2009): 292–93.

Kleinman, Arthur, and Bridget Hanna. "Catastrophe, Caregiving and Today's Biomedicine." *Biosocieties* 3 (2008): 287–301.

Knapp, Clare. "World Report: Health Crisis Worsens in Zimbabwe." *The Lancet* 39 (16 June 2007): 1987–88.

Ko, Dorothy. *Cinderella's Sisters: A Revisionist History of Footbinding*. Berkeley: University of California Press, 2005.

Kohn, Linda T., Janet Corrigan, and Molla S. Donaldson, eds. *To Err Is Human: Building a Safer Health System*. Washington: Institute of Medicine, National Academies Press, 1999.

Kohrman, Matthew, and Xiao Shuiyuan. "Anthropology in China's Health Promotion and Tobacco." *The Lancet* 372.9650 (2008): 1617–18.

Koshy, Rachel C., et al. "Cancer Pain Management in Developing Countries: A Mosaic of Complex Issues Resulting in Inadequate Analgesia." *Supportive Care in Cancer* 6 (1998): 430–37.

Krakauer, Eric. "Just Palliative Care: Responding Responsibly to the Suffering of the Poor." *Journal of Pain and Symptom Management* 36.2 (November 2008): 505–12.

Kuper, Hilda. "The Colonial Situation in Southern Africa." *Journal of Modern African Studies* 2.2 (July 1964): 149–64.

Lakoff, Andrew. "The Generic Biothreat, or, How We Became Unprepared." *Cultural Anthropology* 23.3 (2008): 399–428.

———. "Two Regimes of Global Health." *Humanity: An International Journal of Human Rights, Humanitarianism, and Development* 1.1 (fall 2010): 59–79.

Landau, Paul. "Explaining Surgical Evangelism in Colonial Southern Africa: Teeth, Pain and Faith." *Journal of African History* 37 (1996): 262–81.

Langwick, Stacey. *Bodies, Politics, and African Healing: The Matter of Maladies in Tanzania*. Bloomington: Indiana University Press, 2011.

―――. "Devils, Parasites, and Fierce Needles: Healing and the Politics of Translation in Southern Tanzania." *Science, Technology, and Human Values* 32.1 (2007): 88–117.

Larkin, Brian. *Signal and Noise: Media, Infrastructure, and Urban Culture in Nigeria*. Durham: Duke University Press, 2008.

Lavi, Shai. *The Modern Art of Dying: A History of Euthanasia in the United States*. Princeton: Princeton University Press, 2005.

Lawler, Kathy, et al. "Depression among HIV-Positive Individuals in Botswana: A Behavioral Surveillance." *AIDS and Behavior* 15.1 (2011): 204–8.

Levy, L. M. "Communicating with the Cancer Patient in Zimbabwe." *Communication with the Cancer Patient: Information and Truth*, ed. Antonella Surbone and Matjaz Zwitter, 133–41. New York: New York Academy of Sciences, 1997.

Lingwood, Rebecca J., et al. "The Challenge of Cancer Control in Africa." *Nature Reviews Cancer* 8 (2008): 398–403.

Livingston, Julie. "AIDS as Chronic Illness: Epidemiological Transition and Health Care in Southeastern Botswana." *African Journal of AIDS Research* 3.1 (2004): 15–22.

―――. *Debility and the Moral Imagination in Botswana*. Bloomington: Indiana University Press, 2005.

―――. "Disgust, Bodily Aesthetics, and the Ethic of Being Human in Botswana." *Africa* 78.2 (2008): 288–307.

―――. "Suicide, Risk, and Investment at the Heart of the African Miracle." *Cultural Anthropology* 24.4 (2009): 652–80.

Livingston, Julie, Keith Wailoo, and Barbara Cooper. "HPV Skepticism and Vaccination as Governance: The U.S. and Africa as a Lens onto the North-South Divide." *The HPV Vaccine and Sexual Risk: Citizens and States at the Crossroads of Cancer Prevention*, ed. Keith Wailoo, Julie Livingston, Stephen Epstein, and Robert Aronowitz, 231–53. Baltimore: Johns Hopkins University Press, 2010.

Livingstone, David. *Missionary Travels and Researches in South Africa*. New York: Harper Brothers, 1858.

Lock, Margaret. "Breast Cancer: Reading the Omens." *Anthropology Today* 14 (1998): 7–16.

―――. *Encounters with Aging: Mythologies of Menopause in North America and Japan*. Berkeley: University of California Press, 1995.

―――. *Twice Dead: Organ Transplantation and the Reinvention of Death*. Berkeley: University of California Press, 2001.

Lock, Margaret, and Vinh-Kim Nguyen. *An Anthropology of Biomedicine*. Chichester, UK: Wiley Blackwell, 2010.

Logie, Dorothy, and Mhoira Leng. "Africans Die in Pain because of Fears of Opiate Addiction." *British Medical Journal* 335 (6 October 2007): 685.

Long, Debi, Cynthia L. Hunter, and Sjaak Van der Geest. "Introduction: When the Field Is a Ward or Clinic: Hospital Ethnography." *Anthropology and Medicine* 15.2 (2008): 71–78.

Loram, Charles T. *The Education of the South African Native*. London: Longmans, Green, 1917.

Louie, Karly S., Sylvia de Sanjose, and Philippe Mayaud. "Epidemiology and Prevention of Human Papillomavirus and Cervical Cancer in Sub-Saharan Africa: A Comprehensive Review." *Tropical Medicine and International Health* 14.10 (October 2009): 1287–1302.

Mack, Phyllis. *Heart Religion in the Early Enlightenment: Gender and Emotion in Early Methodism*. New York: Cambridge University Press, 2008.

Maclean, Una. "Nigeria 1956–65: A Medical Memoir." *African Affairs* 83.333 (1984): 543–66.

Macrae, S. M., and B. V. Cook. "A Retrospective Study of the Cancer Patterns among Hospital In-Patients in Botswana, 1960–72." *British Journal of Cancer* 32 (1975): 121–33.

Makoae, Mokhantso. "The Phenomenology of Bodily Care: Caregivers' Experiences with AIDS Patients before Antiretroviral Therapies in Lesotho." *African Journal of AIDS Research* 8.1 (2009): 17–27.

Manyere, Irene. "The Uses of the Pain Assessment Tools by Nurses in Botswana in Assessing and Managing Pain." BEd Nursing thesis, University of Botswana, 1996.

Markowitz, Gerald, and David Rosner. *Deceit and Denial: The Deadly Politics of Industrial Pollution*. Berkeley: University of California Press / Milbank Memorial Fund, 2002.

Martin, Emily. *Flexible Bodies: The Role of Immunity in American Culture from the Days of Polio to the Age of AIDS*. Boston: Beacon, 1994.

McCulloch, Joch. *Asbestos Blues: Labor, Capital, Physicians, and the State in South Africa*. London: James Currey, 2002.

McKenzie, Erin N. Kobetz, James Hnatyszyn, Leo B. Twiggs, and Joseph A. Lucci III. "Women with HIV Are More Commonly Infected with Non-16 and -18 High-Risk HPV Types." *Gynecologic Oncology* 116 (2010): 572–77.

Merriweather, Alfred. *Desert Doctor: Medicine and Evangelism in the Kalahari Desert*. Cambridge: Lutterworth Press, 1969.

———. *Desert Doctor Remembers: The Autobiography of Alfred Merriweather*. Gaborone: Pula Press, 1999.

Miller, William Ian. *The Anatomy of Disgust*. Cambridge: Harvard University Press, 1998.

Milmo, Cahal. "Dumped in Africa: Britain's Toxic Waste." *Independent*, 18 February 2009, http://www.independent.co.uk.

Miyakazi, Hirokazu. *The Method of Hope: Anthropology, Philosophy, and Fijian Knowledge*. Palo Alto: Stanford University Press, 2004.

Mogae, Festus. "State of the Nation Address by His Excellency Mr. Festus G. Mogae, President of the Republic of Botswana to the First Meeting of the Third Session of the Eighth Parliament." 29 October 2001.

Mol, Annemarie. *The Body Multiple: Ontology in Medical Practice*. Durham: Duke University Press, 2002.

———. *The Logic of Care: Health and the Problem of Patient Choice*. New York: Routledge, 2008.

Morris, Kelly. "Cancer? In Africa?" *The Lancet Oncology* 4 (January 2003): 5.

Mosweunyane, Tjantilili. "The Knowledge of Nurses working in Botswana Health Care Settings in Regard to Pain Control." BEd Nursing thesis, University of Botswana, 1994.

Moyo, J. M. "The Extent to which Nurses Meet Clients' Needs for Pain Management within the First 48 Hours Post C-Section." BEd Nursing thesis, University of Botswana, 1994.

"Mpilo General Surgical Centre Shut Down." *Mthwakazian*, 14 December 2010, http://www.mthwakazian.com.

Mukherjee, Siddhartha. *The Emperor of All Maladies: A Biography of Cancer*. New York: Scribner, 2010.

Mulemi, Benson A. "Coping with Cancer and Adversity: Hospital Ethnography in Kenya." PhD diss., University of Amsterdam, 2010.

———. "Patients' Perspectives on Hospitalization: Experiences from a Cancer Ward in Kenya." "Hospital Ethnography," special issue of *Anthropology and Medicine* 15.2 (2008): 117–31.

Mumford, W. B., and C. E. Smith. "Racial Comparisons and Intelligence Testing." *Journal of Royal African Society* 37.146 (January 1938): 46–57.

Muñoz, Nubia, et al. "Epidemiological Classification of Human Papillomavirus Types Associated with Cervical Cancer." *New England Journal of Medicine* 348 (2003): 518–27.

Murphy, Michelle. *Sick Building Syndrome and the Problem of Uncertainty: Environmental Politics, Technoscience, and Women Workers*. Durham: Duke University Press, 2006.

Murphy, Robert. *The Body Silent*. New York: Norton, 1987.

Murray, Scott A., Elizabeth Grant, Angus Grant, and Marilyn Kendall. "Dying from Cancer in Developed and Developing Countries: Lessons from Two Qualitative Interview Studies of Patients and Their Carers." *British Medical Journal* 326 (15 February 2003): 368–71.

Musisi, Nakanyike. "The Politics of Perception or Perception as Politics? Colonial and Missionary Representations of Baganda Women, 1900–1945." *Women in African Colonial Histories*, ed. Jean Allman, Susan Geiger, and Nakanyike Musisi, 95–115. Bloomington: Indiana University Press, 2002.

Mutizwa-Mangiza, Dorothy. *Doctors and the State: The Struggle for Professional Control in Zimbabwe*. London: Ashgate, 1999.

National Cancer Institute, Office of HIV and AIDS Malignancy. "AIDS Malignancy Consortium." http://oham.cancer.gov/.

Ndlovu, Nqobani. "Mpilo Doctors Revolt over 'Appalling Work Conditions.'" *Standard*, 12 November 2006, http://www.thestandard.co.zw.

Ngoma, T. "World Health Organization Cancer Priorities in Developing Countries." *Annals of Oncology* 17, supplement 8 (2006): viii9–viii14.

Nguyen, Vinh-Kim. "Government by Exception: Enrollment and Experimentality in Mass HIV Treatment Programmes in Africa." *Social Theory and Health* 7.3 (2009): 196–217.

———. *The Republic of Therapy: Triage and Sovereignty in West Africa's Time of AIDS*. Durham: Duke University Press, 2010.

Ngwenya, B. N., and B. M. Butale. "HIV/AIDS, Intra-family Resource Capacity and Home Care in Maun." *Botswana Notes and Records* 37 (2005): 138–60.

Nofal, M., F. Durosinmi-Etti, G. P. Hanson, and J. Stjernsward. "Supporting Cancer Care in the Developing Countries: Role of IAEA/WHO." *International Journal of Radiation Oncology, Biology, Physics* 19 (1990): 1249–56.

Nussbaum, Martha. *Hiding from Humanity: Disgust, Shame, and the Law*. Princeton: Princeton University Press, 2006.

Nyamnjoh, Francis. *Insiders and Outsiders: Citizenship and Xenophobia in Contemporary Southern Africa*. London: Zed, 2006.

Nyati-Ramahobo, Lydia. "From a Phone Call to the High Court: Wayeyi Visibility and the Kamanakao Association's Campaign for Linguistic and Cultural Rights in Botswana." *Journal of Southern African Studies* 28.4 (December 2002): 685–709.

Okeke, Iruka. *Divining without Seeds: The Case for Strengthening Laboratory Medicine in Africa*. Ithaca: Cornell University Press, 2011.

Olweny, C. L. M., T. Toya, E. Katongole-Mbidde, J. Mugerwa, S. K. Kyalwazi, and H. Cohen. "Treatment of Hepatocellular Carcinoma with Adriamycin: Preliminary Communication." *Cancer* 36 (1975): 1250–57.

Packard, Randall. "The Healthy Reserve and the Dressed Native: Discourses on Black Health and the Language of Legitimation in Africa." *American Ethnologist* 16.4 (1989): 686–703.

———. "Visions of Postwar Health and Development and Their Impact on Public Health Interventions in the Developing World." *International Development and the Social Sciences*, ed. F. Cooper and R. M. Packard, 93–118. Berkeley: University of California Press, 1997.

———. *White Plague, Black Labor: Tuberculosis and the Political Economy of Health and Disease in South Africa*. Berkeley: University of California Press, 1989.

Packard, Randall, and Paul Epstein. "Epidemiologists, Social Scientists and the Structure of Medical Research on AIDS in Africa." *Social Science and Medicine* 33 (1991): 771–94.

Parkin, D. Max, Freddie Bray, J. Ferlay, and Paola Pisani. "Global Cancer Statistics, 2002." *CA: A Cancer Journal for Clinicians* 55 (2005): 74–108.

Parkin, D. Max, Freddy Sitas, Mike Chirenje, Lara Stein, Raymond Abratt, and Henry Waibinga. "Part 1. Cancer in Indigenous Africans: Burden, Distribution, and Trends." *The Lancet Oncology* 9 (July 2008): 683–92.

Pederson, Susan. "National Bodies, Unspeakable Acts: The Sexual Politics of Colonial Policymaking." *Journal of Modern History* 63.4 (1991): 647–80.

Pellow, David Naguib. *Resisting Global Toxics: Transnational Movements for Environmental Justice.* Cambridge: Massachusetts Institute of Technology Press, 2008.

Pernick, Martin. *A Calculus of Suffering: Pain, Professionalism, and Anesthesia in Nineteenth-Century America.* New York: Columbia University Press, 1985.

Peterson, Kristin. "On the Monopoly: The Changing Nature of Markets and Property in Nigeria and Beyond." Unpublished manuscript.

Petryna, Adriana. *Life Exposed: Biological Citizens after Chernobyl.* Princeton: Princeton University Press, 2002.

———. *When Experiments Travel: Clinical Trials and the Global Search for Human Subjects.* Princeton: Princeton University Press, 2009.

Pettypiece, Shannon. "Global: Merck Gives $500 Million of Vaccine to Poorer Nations." *Bloomberg News*, 24 September 2009, http://www.aegis.com.

Phillips, Richard Cobden. "The Lower Congo: A Sociological Study." *Journal of the Anthropological Institute of Great Britain and Ireland* 17 (1888): 214–37.

Pigg, Stacy Leigh. "Globalizing the Facts of Life." *Sex in Development: Science, Sexuality, and Morality in Global Perspective*, ed. Vincanne Adams and Stacy Leigh Pigg, 39–65. Durham: Duke University Press, 2005.

Portenoy, R., and P. Lesage. "Management of Cancer Pain." *The Lancet* 353.9165 (1999): 1695–1700.

Prentice, Rachel. *Bodies of Information: An Ethnography of Anatomy and Surgery Education.* Durham: Duke University Press, forthcoming.

Price, Elizabeth Lees Moffat. *Journals Written in Bechuanaland, Southern Africa, 1854–1883. With an Epilogue: 1889–1900.* London: E. Arnold, 1956.

"Princess Marina Wards Stink." *Botswana Daily News*, 4 October 2000, http://www.dailynews.gov.bw.

Proctor, Robert. *Cancer Wars: How Politics Shape What We Know and Don't Know about Cancer.* New York: Basic Books, 1996.

Ramiah, Ilavenil, and Michael Reich. "Building Effective Public-Private Partnerships: Experiences and Lessons from the African Comprehensive HIV/AIDS Partnerships (ACHAP)." *Social Science and Medicine* 63.2 (July 2006): 397–408.

Ramogola-Masire, Doreen. "Cervical Cancer, HIV and the HPV Vaccine in Botswana." *The HPV Vaccine and Sexual Risk: Citizens and States at the Crossroads of Cancer Prevention*, ed. Keith Wailoo, Julie Livingston, Stephen Epstein, and Robert Aronowitz, 91–102. Baltimore: Johns Hopkins University Press, 2010.

Rieff, David. *Swimming in a Sea of Death: A Son's Memoir.* New York: Simon and Schuster, 2008.

Roche, Harriet. *On Trek in the Transvaal: Or, Over the Berg and Veldt in South Africa.* London: S. Low, Marston, Seale and Rivington, 1878.

Rosner, David, and Gerald Markowitz. *Deadly Dust, Silicosis and the Struggle for Workers' Health.* Princeton: Princeton University Press, 1991.

Rouse, Carolyn. *Uncertain Suffering: Racial Health Care Disparities and Sickle Cell Disease.* Berkeley: University of California Press, 2009.

Sadowsky, Jonathan. *Imperial Bedlam: Institutions of Madness in Colonial Southwest Nigeria*. Berkeley: University of California Press, 1999.

Sahasrabuddhe, V. V. "Prevalence and Distribution of HPV Genotypes among HIV-infected Women in Zambia." *British Journal of Cancer* 96 (2007): 1480–83.

Sasco, Annie. "From the International Union Against Cancer. Africa: A Desperate Need for Data." *Tobacco Control* 3.3 (1994): 281.

Scarry, Elaine. *The Body in Pain: The Making and Unmaking of the World*. Oxford: Oxford University Press, 1985.

Schapera, Isaac. *Bogwera: Kgatla Initiation*. Pamphlet. Mochudi: Phutadikobo Museum, 1978.

————. *Migrant Labour and Tribal Life: A Study of Conditions in the Bechuanaland Protectorate*. London: Oxford University Press, 1947.

Seligman, C. G. "Anthropological Perspective and Psychological Theory." *Journal of the Royal Anthropological Institute of Great Britain and Ireland* 62 (July 1932): 193–228.

Shiels, Meredith S., et al. "Cancer Burden in the HIV-Infected Population in the United States." *Journal of the National Cancer Institute* 103 (2011): 753–62.

Shouten, Jeffrey. "The Rise and Fall of the AIDS Malignancy Consortium." *Research Initiative Treatment Action* (summer 2003): 30–31.

Sloan, F. A., and H. Gelband, eds. *Cancer Control Opportunities in Low- and Middle-Income Countries*. Washington: Institute of Medicine and the National Academies, National Academies Press, 2007.

Sloley, Herbert. "The African Native Labour Contingent and the Welfare Committee." *Journal of the Royal African Society* 17.67 (April 1918): 199–211.

Smuts, J. C. "Native Policy in Africa." *Journal of the Royal Africa Society* 29.115 (April 1930): 248–68.

Solanke, Toriola F. "Communication with the Cancer Patient in Nigeria." *Communication with the Cancer Patient: Information and Truth*, ed. Antonella Surbone and Matjaz Zwitter, 109–18. New York: New York Academy of Sciences, 1997.

Solway, Jacqueline. "Human Rights and NGO 'Wrongs': Conflict Diamonds, Culture Wars, and the 'Bushman Question.'" *Africa* 80.3 (2009): 321–46.

Songolo, P., E. Chokuonga, S. Motlogi, and L. Mogorsakgomo. *Botswana National Cancer Registry Report, 1986–2004*. Community Health Services Division, Epidemiology and Disease Control Unit, Non-Communicable Diseases Programme, Ministry of Health, Gaborone: Republic of Botswana, 2005.

Stewart, Bernard, and Paul Kleihues, eds. *World Cancer Report*. Lyon: International Agency for Research on Cancer Press, 2003.

Stoneham, H. F. "Origin of Cruelty." *Man* 32 (October 1932): 248.

Sussman, Steve, et al. "Tobacco Control in Developing Countries: Tanzania, Nepal, China, and Thailand as Examples." *Nicotine and Tobacco Research* 9, suppl. 3 (November 2007): S447–57.

"Syphilis in the Uganda Protectorate." *British Medical Journal* 2 (1908): 1037.

"Syphilis in Uganda." *The Lancet* 2 (1908): 1022–23.

Taylor, J. F., A. C. Templeton, C. L. Vogel, J. L. Ziegler, and S. K. Kyalwazi. "Kaposi's Sarcoma in Uganda: A Clinico-pathological Study." *International Journal of Cancer* 8 (1971): 122–35.

Thomas, Lynn. *The Politics of the Womb: Women, Reproduction, and the State in Kenya.* Berkeley: University of California Press, 2003.

Thomson, Joseph. "Journey of the Society's East African Expedition." *Proceedings of the Royal Geographic Society and Monthly Record of Geography*, New Monthly Series 2.12 (December 1880): 721–40.

Thupayagale-Tshweneagae, G. "Migration of Nurses: Is There Any Other Option?" *International Nursing Review* 54 (2007): 107–9.

Travis, Kate. "Cancer in Africa: Health Experts Aim to Curb Potential Epidemic." *Journal of the National Cancer Institute* 99.15 (2007): 1146–47.

Tronto, Joan. *Moral Boundaries: A Political Argument for an Ethic of Care.* New York: Routledge, 1993.

Turshen, Meredeth. *Privatizing Health Services in Africa.* New Brunswick: Rutgers University Press, 1999.

University of Wisconsin Pain and Policy Studies Group. *Availability of Morphine and Pethidine in the World and Africa*, http://www.painpolicy.wisc.edu.

Van Allen, Judith. "'Bad Future Things' and Liberatory Moments: Capitalism, Gender, and the State in Botswana." *Radical History Review* 76 (2000): 136–68.

Van der Geest, Sjaak, and Kaja Finkler. "Hospital Ethnography: Introduction." *Social Science and Medicine* 59.10 (2004): 1995–2001.

Vaughan, Megan. *Curing Their Ills: Colonial Power and African Illness.* Stanford: Stanford University Press, 1991.

———. *Story of an African Famine: Gender and Famine in Twentieth Century Malawi.* Cambridge: Cambridge University Press, 1987.

———. "Syphilis and Sexuality: The Limits of Colonial Medical Power." *Curing Their Ills*, 129–54. Stanford: Stanford University Press, 1991.

Vogel, C. L., C. J. Templeton, A. C. Templeton, J. F. Taylor, and S. K. Kyalwazi. "Treatment of Kaposi's Sarcoma with Actinomycin-D and Cyclophosphamide: Results of a Randomized Clinical Trial." *International Journal of Cancer* 8 (1971): 136–43.

Wailoo, Keith. *How Cancer Crossed the Color Line.* New York: Oxford University Press, 2011.

Wailoo, Keith, and Stephen Pemberton. *The Troubled Dream of Genetic Medicine: Ethnicity and Innovation in Tay-Sachs, Cystic Fibrosis, and Sickle Cell Disease.* Baltimore: Johns Hopkins University Press, 2006.

Wainana, Binyavanga. "How to Write about Africa." *Granta* 92 (winter 2005): 92–94.

Wall, S. R., et al. "Cervical Human Papillomavirus Infection and Squamous Intra-epithelial Lesions in Rural Gambia, West Africa: Viral Sequence Analysis and Epidemiology." *British Journal of Cancer* 93 (2005): 1068–76.

Warren, Chris. *Brush with Death: A Social History of Lead Poisoning.* Baltimore: Johns Hopkins University Press, 2001.

Wendland, Claire. *A Heart for the Work: Journeys through an African Medical School.* Chicago: University of Chicago Press, 2010.

Werbner, Richard, ed. "Challenging Minorities, Differences, and Tribal Citizenship in Botswana." Special issue of *Journal of Southern African Studies* 28.4 (2002).

——. *Holy Hustlers, Schism, and Prophecy: Apostolic Reformation in Botswana.* Berkeley: University of California Press, 2011.

Whyte, Susan Reynolds. *Questioning Misfortune: The Pragmatics of Uncertainty in Eastern Uganda.* Cambridge: Cambridge University Press, 1997.

Whyte, Susan Reynolds, Michael Whyte, and David Kyaddondo. "Health Workers Entangled: Confidentiality and Certification." *Morality, Hope and Grief: Anthropologies of AIDS in Africa*, ed. Hansjoerg Dilger and Uta Luig, 80–101. New York: Berghahn, 2010.

Whyte, Susan Reynolds, Michael Whyte, Lotte Meinart, and Betty Kyaddondo. "Treating AIDS: Dilemmas of Unequal Access in Uganda." *SAHARA-J: Journal of Social Aspects of HIV/AIDS* 1.1 (2004): 14–26.

Williams, A. Olufemi, and Gregory T. O'Connor. "Introduction." *Virus-Associated Cancers in Africa*, ed. A. Olufemi Williams, Gregory T. O'Connor, Guy B. De-The, and Couavi A. Johnson, xiii–xiv. Lyon: Oxford University Press, 1984.

Williams, A. Olufemi, Gregory T. O'Connor, Guy B. De-The, and Couavi A. Johnson, eds. *Virus-Associated Cancers in Africa.* Lyon: Oxford University Press, 1984.

Willoughby, W. C. "Notes on the Initiation Ceremonies of the Becwana." *Journal of the Royal Anthropological Institute of Great Britain and Ireland* 39 (1909): 228–45.

Wind, Gitte. "Negotiated Interactive Observation: Doing Fieldwork in Hospital Settings." *Anthropology and Medicine* 15.2 (2008): 79–89.

Wood, J. G. *The Uncivilized Races of Men in all Countries of the World.* Vol. 1. San Francisco: J. A. Brainard, 1882.

Woodworth, R. S. "Racial Differences in Mental Traits." *Science* 31.788 (February 1910): 177.

World Health Organization. "Cholera in Zimbabwe: Epidemiological Bulletin Number 24, Week 21 (17–23 May 2009)." World Health Organization, http://www.who.int.

——. *A Community Health Approach to Palliative Care for HIV/AIDS and Cancer Patients.* Geneva: World Health Organization, 2003.

——. *Tobacco Atlas 2002.* World Health Organization, http://www.who.int.

Ziegler, J. L., M. H. Cohen, R. H. Morrow, S. K. Kyalwazi, and P. P. Carbone. "Immunologic Studies in Burkitt's Lymphoma." *Cancer* 25 (1970): 734–39.

"Zimbabwe: Recession Hits Renal Patients." IRIN Humanitarian News and Analysis, 1 October 2007, http://www.irinnews.org.

Zoborowski, Mark. *People in Pain.* San Francisco: Jossey-Bass, 1969.